SIRTFOOD DIET COOKBOOK

200 Healthy, Easy-To-Make and Tasty Recipes to Lose Weight Fast and Improve YOUR Life. An Easy-To-Follow 21-Day Plan to Burn Fat and Enjoy YOUR Life Feeling Great and Healthy.

GEENA MOORE

DISCLAIMER

This book is meant for educational and information purposes only. It is not meant to give any medical advice, diagnose, or treat any medical conditions. No medical claims are made in this book. The nutritional advice given in this book will not treat or cure medical conditions, metabolic disorders, or other illnesses. The nutritional advice is meant for healthy individuals who want to improve their appearance for cosmetic reasons and not to treat illnesses of any kind.

You should always consult your physician or other healthcare provider should you have any questions regarding a medical condition or treatment plan.

The author is not a MD or RD and cannot be held liable or responsible to any person or entity with respect to any information contained in this book. The reader/ user assumes all risks for any injury, loss or damage caused or alleged to be caused directly or indirectly by using the information contained in this book.

Table of Contents

Introduction

So, you are ready to lose weight, but you are not sure how. You are looking through diets online. You see the Mediterranean Diet. You see the Keto Diet. You see the Paleo Diet. There are countless options out there, all touting that they are the best because they will help you to lose weight quickly. Which one do you choose? You may scroll through them all without choosing one that seems right for you because you cannot think of one that is just right. You see all sorts of options, but none of them call out. Maybe you've tried Keto, but you missed your fruits and carbs too much. Perhaps you tried the Paleo diet, but it just was not doing it for you. Whether you have failed a diet in the past does not have to define the future for you; however—you can lose weight. You can learn how you can properly shed it off so that you will be able to love your own skin and stay healthier. Perhaps you just need a new way of making it work for you.

The Sirtfood Diet is a new diet that was designed in the UK, created by celebrity nutritionists, Aidan Goggins and Glen Matten, and published in a recipe book in 2016. Designed to allow for you to eat certain foods that will allow you to trigger your skinny gene, the diet is designed to help people rapidly shed the pounds without the same consequences that are commonly seen in other fad diets. Some diets require you to starve yourself and wind up, causing loss of muscle along with the fat. Others require you to give up on foods that you enjoy, making them so restrictive that they are difficult for most people to keep up with. However, the Sirtfood Diet encourages you to focus on sirtuin-rich foods that can be combined into meals that are delicious and satisfying. How does chicken curry sound? You can consume it on the Sirtfood Diet. What about a nice turmeric salmon? That is also a meal that you can enjoy. You can even enjoy blueberry pancakes for breakfast on this diet as well.

We are going to take a look at the Sirtfood Diet. We are going to address what it is and whether it is effective. Finally, we will take a look at whether this diet is going to be right for you in the long run. This diet will involve phases of dieting, which will sometimes have you restricting calories down to 1000 per day, and that is not always safe for all people. However, if this diet is right for you, you will find that this could be a great option for you. Even if you cannot fully follow the diet, just enjoying these foods that are rich in sirtuins is a great way to support your diet and add all sorts of healthy foods to the mix.

Scientists have found that sirtuins play a critical role in weight loss, arranging the cellulose and, most importantly, restructuring the muscles in the body. There is ongoing research on this subject. Research has also found that humans have seven sirtuins and if they can activate some of it, it could help burn fat and treat obesity and diabetes. This proposition further states that the effectiveness of sirtuins displaces the need to follow other diets or physical exercise.

With constant reports of deaths resulting from chronic illnesses, the importance of a sirtfood diet intake is further brought to light. Excess fat is said to clot the blood cells and to be capable of leading to death as a result. The sirtfood diet can avert this by igniting loss of unwanted fat. However, it takes considerable sacrifice to achieve this.

Chapter 1:   What Is a Sirtfood?

The sirtfood diet was created by British nutritionists Aidan Goggins and Glen Matten, who are distributing a book with a top score in 2016. It promises to reduce irritation, extend its shelf life, activate "good quality," and help you shed seven pounds (three pounds) in seven days. He argues that the consumption of certain foods will interact with a collection of proteins found in the body called sirtuins (sirtuins), which are involved in a wide range of cellular forms such as digestion, maturation, and the circadian rhythm.

In addition to expanding the reach of "sirtfoods," the diet includes phases of calorie restriction, which are also said to allow the body to produce more sirtuins. During the first three, they say that the calorie intake is limited to 1,000 each day, from three green juices and a dinner rich in sirtfood. For the rest of the week, calorie intake is aided by 1,500 daily of two juices and two dinners. In the long run, his supporters propose eating dinners with as many sirt foods as reasonably expected.

There are many sirtuin-activating foods to choose from, some contain more ingredients that activate sirtuin than others. We have called them "the best sirtfood foods," and these foods are included in all of our recipes to maximize your sirt food intake.

It has become one of the most popular names in Europe and is popular for its red wine and chocolate licenses.

Its manufacturers claim that it is nothing more than a frequent fad, but instead of "sirtfoods," it is the key to opening misfortune and preventing disease.

In any case, wellness experts warn that this diet may not meet everyone's expectations and may even be a misunderstanding.

Two VIP nutritionists working for a private discovery center in the UK have created the sirtfood diet.

They publish the diet plan as a new progressive diet and wellness program that works by activating its "good quality."

This treatment relies on research into sirtuins (sirtuins), a concentration of seven proteins found in the body, and appears to handle a variety of possibilities, including digestion, irritation, and life expectancy, some characteristic plant mixtures may have the option to increase the degree of these proteins in the body and the nutrients they have called "sirtfoods."

The sirtfood diet depends on the examination of sirtuins, a concentration of protein that directs some abilities in the body. Some foods called sirtfoods can cause the body to make more of these proteins.

Benefits Of Sirt Food Nutrition

The Sirtfood diet depends on a new collection of foods called Sirtfoods. These wonderful nutrients in the body will activate an impressive reuse cycle that eliminates cellular waste and absorbs fat. Everything they do taking our sirtuin properties also called "thin" conditions. These are similar properties applied by exercise and fasting.

Top Sirtfoods incorporate

Pecans	Green tea	Red onions	Cocoa
Parsley	Additional	Strawberries	Curry Flavors

	Virgin olive oil		
Espresso	Kale	Rocket	

Unlike recently advanced diets where the emphasis is on nutrition elimination, with Sirtfoods, the benefits are given by eating.

Preliminary members in our Sirtfood Diet lost an amazing 7 pounds over the underlying seven days, remembering increments for muscle and muscle work. This dramatic impact on fat-consuming, while muscle progression, is one reason that our Sirtfood-based diet has gotten so well-known with anybody needing to get slender and fit as a fiddle, much the same as the world-class competitors and models. They have supported this way of eating.

However, to consider it absolutely as a weight reduction diet is to overlook the main issue. This is a diet that has a lot to do with wellbeing as waistlines. Expanded vitality, brighter skin, feeling alarmed progressively, and better rest is the beautiful 'reactions' from along these lines of eating. Once in a while, the advantages are significantly increasingly momentous, remembering situations where following the diet for the more extended term has turned around metabolic ailments

The main concern is evident: If you need to accomplish a progressively vivacious, slenderer, and healthier body, and establish the frameworks for deep-rooted health and protection from the ailment, at that point, the Sirtfood Diet is for you.

Can You Eat Meat on Sirtfood?

The diet plan not just incorporates expending a good part of the meat, it suggests that protein be a primary consideration in a Sirtfood-based diet to receive the greatest reward in keeping up digestion and reducing the muscle exhaustion necessary in most diet plans. It is anything but a meat-overwhelming food (we despite everything recall the terrible breath from the Atkins diet), it's in reality very veggie-lover well-disposed and caters for practically everybody, which is the thing that makes it so reasonable an alternative.

Leucine is an amino corrosive found in protein, which supplements and improves the activities of Sirtfoods. This implies the ideal approach to eat Sirtfoods is by consolidating them with a chicken breast, steak, or another wellspring of leucine, for example, fish or eggs.

Poultry can be eaten uninhibitedly (because it is an excellent wellspring of protein, B nutrients, potassium, and phosphorous). That red meat (another fantastic wellspring of protein, iron, zinc, and nutrient B12) can be eaten up to multiple times (750g crude weight) seven days.

"Sirtfood" seems like something created by outsiders, brought to earth for human utilization with expectations of picking up mind control and global control. Sirt foods are foods high in sirtuins. Uh, come back once more?

How can it work?

At its center, the way to getting in shape is genuinely straightforward: Create a calorie shortfall either by expanding your calorie consumption exercises or diminishing your caloric admission. As it may imagine a scenario where you could skirt the abstaining from excessive food intake and instead activate a "thin quality" without the requirement for extreme calorie limitation. This is the reason for The Sirtfood Diet, composed by nourishment specialists Aidan Goggins and Glen Matten. The best approach to do it, they contend, is Sirt foods.

Sirtfoods are wealthy in supplements that activate an alleged "thin quality" called sirtuin. As indicated by Goggins and Matten, the "thin quality" is activated when a lack of vitality is made after you confine calories. Sirtuins got fascinating to the nourishment world in 2003 when analysts found that resveratrol, a compound found in red wine, had a similar impact on life length as calorie limitation; however, it was accomplished without lessening admission. (Discover the complete truth about wine and its medical advantages.)

In the 2015 pilot study, testing the adequacy of sirtuins, the 39 members lost a normal of seven pounds in seven days. Those outcomes sound amazing. However, it's critical to understand this is a small example size concentrated over a brief timeframe. Weight reduction specialists additionally have their questions about the grandiose guarantees. The cases made are extremely theoretical and extrapolate from considers which were, for the most part, centeredon basic creatures (like yeast) at the cell level. What occurs at the cell level doesn't mean what occurs in the human body at the full-scale level.

What Are the Advantages?

You will get thinner if you follow this eating regimen intently. Regardless of whether you're eating 1,000 calories of tacos, 1,000 calories of kale, or 1,000 calories of snickerdoodles, you will get in shape at 1,000 calories. In any case, she likewise brings up that you can have accomplishments an increasingly sensible calorie limitation. The typical day by day caloric admission of somebody not on a careful nutritional plan is 2,000 to 2,200, so diminishing to 1,500 is as yet confining and would be a viable weight reduction procedure for most.

Medical Advantages of Sirtfood Diet

Sirtfood diet diminishes the danger of heart infections, heftiness, diabetes, and early demise. Individuals who are following this eating regimen plan has encountered a few medical advantages, generally safe of ailment and prosperity. A portion of the regular medical advantages of sirtfood counts calories are as per the following:

- It will assist you with losing fat, not muscles.
- The eating routine won't deplete your vitality and rather keep you increasingly lively.
- As it thoroughly relies upon diet, setting off to the rec center or performing thorough activities is a bit much.
- The eating regimen plan stays away from the self-starvation hypothesis for weight reduction.
- It forestalls various ceaseless illnesses as the nourishments remembered for this eating regimen plan are solid and nutritive.

Who Should Try Sirtfood Diet?

You know that you have overindulged during the holidays, but as you weigh yourself, you literally would want to shave all the extra pounds because you did not expect to have gained that much weight!

There is an upcoming wedding event, and you need to lose those extra pounds in order to fit yourself into your gown/suit. There is no way that you are going to lose that much weight in 2 months!

You know that you are overweight and just plain unhealthy. You have already tried a number of diets but to no avail. Either you feel that those diets are too restrictive, there is an adverse health effect, and the diet is too expensive to maintain. Speaking of maintenance, you have a hard time keeping off the little weight that you have managed to lose!

You are getting older, and you start to notice that aside from having a hard time dealing with hangovers and late-night parties, losing and maintaining weight is not that easy as it used to be. You are not a big fan of eliminating numerous food groups and doing rigorous exercise.

You have probably heard these scenarios too many times before, and you have probably experienced one or two, or you are in one of these scenarios right now. Being overweight or obese Is actually one of the most common health problems around the world. According to the world health organization (who), being overweight is when your BMI is equal to or greater than 25 whiles being obese is when your BMI is equal to or greater than 30 (you can check your BMI here.)

In the 2014 data from who, worldwide obesity has more than doubled since 1980, and more than 1.9 billion adults are overweight; and it would be safe to conclude that after two years that that number has already increased significantly.

Health experts agree that this is a very alarming rate, but the good news is, obesity or having excess weight is preventable and reversible.

As you will notice, most of these scenarios are focused on the aesthetics – looking good and feeling more confident about your body, but what I would like to stress is the ill-effects of every extra bulge or pound that we carry. The possible health illnesses associated with being overweight is the primary reason why you need to try the revolutionary sirtfood diet.

Chapter 2:   Sirtfood Diet Phases

Phase 1: 7 Pounds In Seven Days

Monday: 3 green juices

- Breakfast: water + tea or espresso + a cup of green juice;
- Lunch: green juice
- Snack: a square of dark chocolate;
- Dinner: Sirt meal
- After dinner: a square of dark chocolate.

Drink the juices at three distinct times of the day (for example, in the morning as soon as you wake up, mid-morning and mid-afternoon) and choose the normal or vegan dish: pan-fried oriental prawns with buckwheat spaghetti or miso and tofu with sesame glaze and sautéed vegetables (vegan dish)

Tuesday: 3 green juices

- Breakfast: water + tea or espresso + a cup of green juice
- Lunch: 2 green juices before dinner;
- Snack: a square of dark chocolate;
- Dinner: Sirt meal
- After dinner: a square of dark chocolate.

Welcome to day 2 of the Sirtfood Diet. The formula is identical to that of the first day, and the only thing that changes is the solid meal. Today you will also have dark chocolate, and the same goes for tomorrow. This food is so wonderful that we don't need an excuse to eat it.

To earn the title of a "Sirt food," chocolate must be at least 85 percent cocoa. And even among the various types of chocolate with this percentage, not all of them are the same. This product often is treated with an alkalizing agent (this is the so-called "Dutch process") to reduce its acidity and give it a darker color. Unfortunately, this process greatly reduces the flavonoids activating sirtuins, compromising their health benefits. Lindt Excellence 85% chocolate, is not subjected to the Dutch process and is therefore often recommended.

On day 2, capers are also included in the menu. Despite what many may think, they are not fruits, but buds that grow in Mediterranean countries and are picked by hand. They are fantastic Sirt foods because they are very rich in the nutrients kaempferol and quercetin. From the point of view of flavor, they are tiny concentrates of taste. If you've never used them, don't feel intimidated. You will see, they will taste amazingly if combined with the right ingredients, and they will give an unmistakable and inimitable aroma to your dishes.

On the second day, you will intake: 3 green Sirt juices and one solid meal (normal or vegan).

Drink the juices at three distinct times of the day (for example, when you wake up in the morning, mid-morning and mid-afternoon) and choose either the normal or the vegan dish: Turkey escalope with capers, parsley, and sage on spiced cauliflower couscous or curly kale and red onion Dahl with buckwheat (vegan dish)

Wednesday: 3 green juices

- Breakfast: water + tea or espresso + a cup of green juice
- Lunch: 2 green juices before dinner;
- Snack: a square of dark chocolate;
- Dinner: Sirt meal

- After dinner: a square of dark chocolate.

You are now on the third day, and even if the format is once again identical to that of days 1 and 2, so the time has come to flavor everything with a fundamental ingredient. For thousands of years, chili has been a fundamental element of the gastronomic experiences of the whole world.

As for the effects on health, we have already seen that its spiciness is perfect for activating sirtuins and stimulating the metabolism. The applications of chili are endless, and therefore represent an easy way to consume a Sirt food regularly.

If you are not a big expert of chili, we recommend the Bird's Eye (sometimes called Thai chili), because it is the best for sirtuins.

This is the last day you will consume three green juices a day; tomorrow, you will switch to two. We, therefore, take this opportunity to browse other drinks that you can have during the diet. We all know that green tea is good for health, and water is naturally very good, but what about coffee? More than half of people drink at least one coffee a day, but always with a trace of guilt because some say that it is a vice and an unhealthy habit. This is absolutely untrue; studies show that coffee is a real treasure trove of beneficial plant substances. That's why coffee drinkers run the least risk of getting diabetes, certain forms of cancer, and neurodegenerative diseases. Furthermore, not only is coffee, not a toxin, it protects the liver and makes it even healthier!

Thursday: 2 green juices

- Breakfast: water + tea or espresso + a cup of green juice;
- Lunch: Sirt food;

- Snack: 1 green juice before dinner
- Dinner: Sirtfood

The fourth day of the Sirtfood Diet has arrived, and you are halfway through your journey to a leaner and healthier body. This means that on the fourth day and the upcoming ones, you will have two green juices and two solid meals, all delicious and rich in Sirtfoods. The inclusion of Medjool dates in a list of foods that promote weight loss and good health may seem surprising. Especially when you think they contain 66 percent sugar.

Sugar has no stimulating properties towards sirtuins. On the contrary, it has well-known links with obesity, heart disease, and diabetes; in short, just at the antipodes of the objectives, we aim to. But industrially refined and processed sugar is very different from the sugar present in a food that also contains sirtuin-activating polyphenols: the Medjool dates. Unlike normal sugar, these dates, consumed in moderation, do not increase the level of glucose in the blood.

Friday: 2 green juices

- Breakfast: Water + tea or espresso + a cup of green juice
- Lunch: Sirtfood
- Snack: A green juice before dinner;
- Dinner: Sirtfood

You have reached the fifth day, and the time has come to add fruits. Due to its high sugar content, fruits have been the subject of bad publicity. This does not apply to berries. Strawberries have a very low sugar content: one teaspoon per 100 grams. They also have an excellent effect on how the body processes simple sugars.

Scientists have found that if we add strawberries to simple sugars, this causes a reduction in insulin demand, and therefore transforms food into a machine that releases energy for a long time. Strawberries are, therefore, a perfect element in diets that will help you lose weight and get back in shape. They are also delicious and extremely versatile, as you will discover in the Sirt version of the fresh and light Middle Eastern tabbouleh.

Miso, made from fermented soy, is a traditional Japanese dish. Miso contains a strong umami taste, a real explosion for the taste buds. In our modern society, we know better monosodium glutamate, artificially created to reproduce the same flavor. Needless to say, it is far preferable to derive that magical umami flavor from traditional and natural food, full of beneficial substances. It is found in the form of a paste in all good supermarkets and healthy food stores and should be present in every kitchen to give a touch of taste to many different dishes.

Saturday: 2 green juices

- Breakfast: Water + tea or espresso + a cup of green juice
- Lunch: Sirtfood
- Snack: A green juice before dinner;
- Dinner: Sirtfood

There are no Sirtfood better than olive oil and red wine. Virgin olive oil is obtained from the fruit only by mechanical means, in conditions that do not deteriorate it, so that you can be sure of its quality and polyphenol content. "Extra virgin" oil is that of the first pressing ("virgin" is the result of the second) and therefore has more flavor and better quality: this is what we strongly recommend you to use when cooking.

No Sirt menu would be complete without red wine, one of the cornerstones of the diet. It contains the activators of resveratrol and piceatannol sirtuins, which probably explain the longevity and slenderness associated with the traditional French way of life, and which are at the origin of the enthusiasm unleashed by Sirtfood.

Super lentil Sirt salad (vegan dish) and mole sauce of red beans with roasted potato (vegan dish).

Sunday: 2 green juices

- Breakfast: A bowl of Sirt Muesli + a cup of green juice
- Lunch: Sirtfood
- Snack: A cup of green juice;
- Dinner: Sirtfood

The seventh day is the last of phase 1 of the diet. Instead of considering it as an end, see it as a beginning, because you are about to embark on a new life, in which Sirtfood will play a central role in your nutrition. Today's menu is a perfect example of how easy it is to integrate them in abundance into your daily diet. Just take your favorite dishes and, with a pinch of creativity, you will turn them into a Sirt banquet.

On the seventh day, you will assume 2 green Sirt juices; 2 solid meals (normal or vegan).Drink the juices at different times of the day (for example the first in the morning as soon as you wake up or in the middle of the morning, the second in the middle of the afternoon) and choose the normal or vegan dishes: Sirt omelet Sirt and baked aubergine wedges with walnut and parsley pesto and tomato salad (vegan dish).

During the second phase, there are no calorie restrictions, but indications on which Sirtfood must be eaten to consolidate weight loss and not run the risk of getting the lost kilograms back.

Phase 2: Maintenance

Congratulations! You have finished the first "hardcore" week. The second phase is the easier and is the actual incorporation of sirtuin-filled food selections to your everyday diet or meals. You can call this the "maintenance stage."

By doing so, your body will undergo the fat-burning stage and muscle gain plus a boost on your immune system and overall health.

In this phase, you can now have 3 balanced Sirtfood-filled meals each day plus 1 green juice a day.

There is no "dieting," but more on choosing healthier alternatives with adding Sirtfood in each meal as much as possible.

I will be providing some recipes for tasty dishes with Sirtfood inclusion to further give you an idea of how exciting and healthy this diet journey is.

Now you move back up to a regular calorie intake intending to keep your weight loss steady and your Sirtfood intake high. You should have experienced some degree of weight loss by now, but you should also feel trimmer and re-invigorated.

Phase 2 lasts for 14 days. During this time, you eat 3 sirtfood rich meals, 1 sirtfood green juice, and up to 2 optional Sirtfood bite snacks. Strict calorie-counting is actively discouraged – if you follow the recommendations and eat balanced meals of reasonable portions, you shouldn't feel hungry or be consuming too much.

You should consume the same beverages you were drinking in phase 1, with the slight change that you are welcome to enjoy the occasional glass of red wine (although don't drink more than 3 per week).

Chapter 3:   Shopping List

Ingredients that you should always have at home for the Sirtfood Diet

You should always have the following ingredients at home when you follow the Goggins and mats diet. So, this is your ultimate shopping list:

- Vegetables, fresh
- These vegetables occur almost every day. So always keep it in stock.
- Kale
- Garlic
- Thai chili (Bird's eye chili)
- Red onions
- Beverages
- Black coffee)
- Red wine (Pinot Noir, aka Pinot Noir)
- Tea (green, black, white)
- Water
- Herbs, fresh
- These herbs are used so often that you should always have them fresh at home. It is best to pull them yourself!
- Leaf parsley
- Ginger (even if it's not an herb, let's put it in here...)
- Lovage
- Herbs and spices, dried
- Curry mix; mild, medium or hot to taste
- Coriander
- Cumin (cumin)
- Turmeric

- Sage
- Mustard seeds
- Tamari or Soy sauce
- Nuts
- Walnuts
- Fruit, fresh
- Lemons
- Oils
- Extra virgin olive oil
- Other foods
- Buckwheat
- Chocolate (at least 85% cocoa)

Cooking With Sirtfoods

Now that you have read the list of sirtfoods, it's time to plan your menu so that you can shop for all your required ingredients. If possible, aim to buy your fresh ingredients every few days and include sirtfoods in every meal.

By far, the best way to load up on those sirtfoods is to start your day with a healthy smoothie. Especially a green one as it's a great refreshing kick start to your body and you can easily pack in 5Fruits/vegetables in one drink. It's sure to keep hunger away too!

We've provided lots of recipes for smoothies that you can not only have for breakfast but as a lunch replacement or mid-day snack. Bear in mind that although the recipes have been categorized as breakfast, light bites and main meals, etc.,you are free to swap them around.

If you have had a busy day and haven't been able to pack in the sirt goodies as much as you would like, you can always supplement with a handful of walnuts, a green tea or a coffee in between meals to give you a boost and keep hunger away.

If you are careful with your calorie intake, you can be guided by the information on each recipe. A little word of caution when it comes to dates or 'nature's toffees' as some people call them – they are rich in calories. One date contains around 61 calories, so don't go overboard. That said, if you would normally reach for cakes, sweets or biscuits, then a date or two is a good substitute because you won't be consuming empty refined sugar calories, yet still enjoying a sweet treat.

If you haven't already, swap your normal cuppa for green tea, which has virtually zero calories. If you don't have a taste for it, you can try it with a flavoring such as jasmine, or even try the recipe for iced cranberry green tea for a refreshing way to drink it. Matcha, which is a type of green tea, is an even stronger tea which also comes in a powder that can be added to smoothies and cooking. Health shops stock matcha, or alternatively, you can buy it online.

Keep a parsley plant on your window ledge because you can add it to virtually anything or even nibble on a sprig! Lovage is a relative of parsley, which has even greater sirtuin-activating benefits, so if you can find it (and it's a big if), use that instead of parsley. Because it's not so easy to find, we have not included lovage in any of these recipes, but if you are getting hold of some, just add it in.

Capers are available in most supermarkets and sold in jars. They do have a strong salty flavor so you won't need to use too many.

When it comes to chocolate, don't be tempted to buy a sugar-laden milk chocolate bar at the checkout because it won't contain much cocoa. Always aim for good quality dark chocolate with a high cocoa content of around 85% cocoa.

Yes, it is bitter, but your taste buds will soon adapt, and a square of chocolate after a meal is a great treat to round off the day.

The eating regimen originates from a similar name. The creators – Aidan Goggins and Glen Matten – of the sirtfood diet exhort eating for the most part nourishments rich in sirtuins, a sort of protein in plant nourishments. "The eating plan itself is intended to 'turn on' the sirtuin qualities (especially sirt-1), which are accepted to support digestion, increment fat consuming, battle aggravation, and control craving," says Clark.

Early investigations propose that calorie limitation and resveratrol (a polyphenol found in nourishments like grapes, blueberries, and peanuts), initiate the sirt-1 quality, and these two standards support the sirtfood way to deal with eating.

21 Day Meal Plan

Days	Breakfast	Main meals	Snacks
1	Egg muffins or tortilla, muffins chickpea flour or pure peanut butter meal	Fiesta chicken salad or easy broccoli salad with almond and lemon sauce	Banana slices with peanut butter
2	Egg or Chickpea Muffins Remaining or Peanut Butter Oatmeal	Shrimp with garlic in coconut milk, tomatoes and coriander or zucchini, peas and spinach risotto	Apple with a sunflower/ pumpkin combination
3	Clean eating egg and basil vegetable stir or tofu factory	Remaining taco salad or wild rice Burrito bowl	Celery with peanut butter and raisins
4	Berry oatmeal	Tuna salad with avocado or sliced tofu pesto sandwich	Pieces of cucumber with hummus
5	Sirt Muesli	Tuscan Stewed Beans	Green Egg Scramble
6	Protein pancakes or old vegan pancakes	Orange and almond salad with avocado or fall harvest salad with pomegranate vinaigrette snack:	Pear and peanuts

		popcorn with egg	
7	Hot protein or vegan pancakes	Zucchini pasta with seafood or zucchini pasta with avocado	Baby carrots with guacamole
8	Flourless banana and chocolate pumpkin muffins or raspberry and pumpkin muffins	Chicken and remaining orange salad or orange tofu	Brown rice salad, peanut butter and a tablespoon of honey or maple syrup
9	Apple and bacon sandwich	Toasted grilled salmon with mango sauce or smoked tempeh	Banana and zucchini muffins without chocolate
10	Egg muffins or sun-dried tomato cake.	Bowl of mushrooms and cauliflower	Baked sweet potato with peanut butter, banana and cinnamon
11	Apple and bacon sandwich	Waldorf chicken salad with avocado or vegan Waldorf salad	Cherry or vegan yolks
12	Remains of breakfast yolks or vegan yolks	Banana pieces with vanilla butter and cocoa powder.	Carrots and hummus
13	Breakfast: sweet potato toast	Salad with avocado and shrimp (using the rest of the beans) or sweet	Bony popcorn with hard-boiled eggs or some grilled chickpeas

		and sour tofu	
14	Sweet potato toast	Roasted dry herb and garlic sandwich: Larabar	Pieces of cucumber and hummus
15	Cereals with berries, veal and coconut.	Citrus chicken strips on a spinach salad	Boiled eggs or two roasted chickpeas and carrots with hummus
16	Cereals with berries, veal and coconut.	Citrus chicken strips on a spinach salad	Boiled eggs or two roasted chickpeas and carrots with hummus
17	Oatmeal spices	Vintage chicken salad or lentil cucumber salad	Brown rice with peanut butter and banana piece.
18	Left-over apple spice overnight oats	Left-over harvest chicken salad or lentil cucumber salad	Apple and couple roasted chickpeas
19	Fresh fruit and rice	Greek quinoa salad	Banana and pistachios
20	Black bean scramble or spiced chickpea	Leftovers – green quinoa salad	Chocolate cherry energy bites
21	Banana oat protein muffins	Left-over homemade chicken noodle soup or curried butternut squash soup	Apple chips dipped in peanut butter

Chapter 4: Over 200 Healthy Sirtfood Recipes - Breakfast Recipes

1. Sirt Muesli

Preparation time: 10 minutes

Cooking time: 0 minutes

Serves: 1

Ingredients:

- 0.9-ounce buckwheat flakes
- 0.45 ounce of buckwheat puffs
- 1 ounce of Medjool dates, pitted and chopped
- Walnuts, chopped
- Coconut flakes or desiccated coconut
- 3.5 ounce of strawberries, hulled and chopped
- 0.45 ounce of cocoa nibs
- 3.5 ounce of plain Greek yogurt

Directions:

1. You need to mix the dry ingredients and place them in an airtight container if you want to make it in a large amount or prepare it the night before.

Nutrition:

- Calories: 104,
- Sodium: 33 mg,
- Dietary Fiber: 1.4 g,
- Total Fat: 4.1 g,
- Total Carbs: 16.3 g,
- Protein: 1.3 g.

2. Lamb, Butternut Squash and Date Tagine

Preparation Time: 15 minutes

Cooking time: 40 minutes

Servings: 4 to 6

Ingredients:

- 2 tablespoons olive oil
- 2cm ginger, grated
- 1 red onion, sliced
- 3 garlic cloves, grated or crushed
- 1 teaspoon chili flake (or to taste)
- 1 cinnamon stick
- 2 teaspoons cumin seeds
- 2 teaspoons ground turmeric
- ½ teaspoon salt
- Lamb neck fillet, cut into 2cm chunks
- Medjool dates, pitted and chopped
- 14 ounces of tin chopped tomatoes, plus half a can of water
- 14 ounces of tin chickpeas, drained
- 15.5 ounces of butternut squash, cut into 1cm cubes
- 2 tablespoons fresh coriander (plus extra for garnish)
- Buckwheat, couscous, flatbreads or rice to serve

Directions:

1. Preheat the oven until 140C.
2. Sprinkle about two tablespoons of olive oil in a large oven-proof casserole dish or cast-iron pot. Put the sliced onion and cook on a gentle heat until the onions softened but not brown, with the lid on for about 5 minutes.
3. Add chili, cumin, cinnamon and turmeric to the grated garlic and ginger. Remove well, and cook the lid off for one more minute. If it gets too dry, add a drop of water.

4. Add pieces of lamb. In the onions and spices, stir well to coat the meat and then add salt, chopped dates and tomatoes, plus about half a can of water (100- 200ml).
5. Bring the tagine to the boil, then put the lid on and put it for 1 hour and 15 minutes in your preheated oven.
6. Add the chopped butternut squash and drained chickpeas thirty minutes before the end of the cooking time. Stir all together, bring the lid back on and go back to the oven for the remaining 30 minutes of cooking.
7. Remove from the oven when the tagine is finished, and stir through the chopped coriander. Serve with couscous, buckwheat, flatbreads, or basmati rice.

Notes:

If you don't own an oven-proof casserole dish or cast-iron casserole, cook the taginc in a regular casserole until it has to go into the oven and then transfer the tagine to a regular lidded casserole dish before placing it in the oven. Add 5 minutes of cooking time to provide enough time to heat the casserole dish.

Nutrition:

- Calories: 104,
- Sodium: 33 mg,
- Dietary Fiber: 1.4 g,
- Total Fat: 4.1 g,
- Total Carbs: 16.3 g,
- Protein: 1.3 g.

3. Chicken With Kale, Red Onions and Chili Salsa

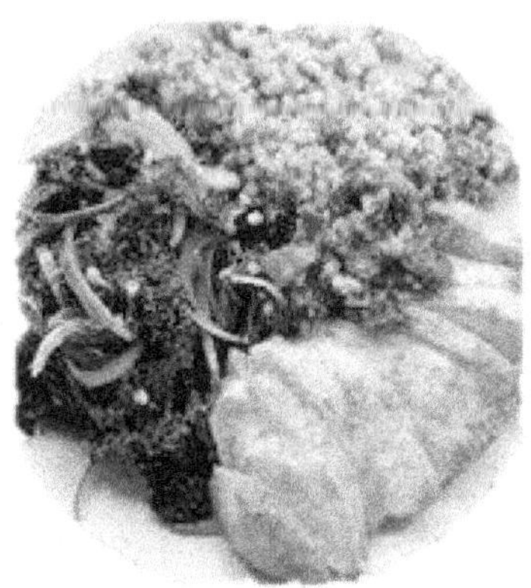

Preparation time: 5 Minutes

Cooking Time: 70 Minutes

Servings: 2

Ingredients:

For the salsa:

- 130g tomatoes
- 1 Thai chilies, finely chopped
- 1 tablespoon capers, finely chopped
- 5 g parsley, finely chopped
- Juice of a quarter of a lemon
- For the rest:
- 3 ounces of chicken breast
- 2 teaspoons turmeric
- Juice of a quarter of a lemon
- 1 tablespoon of olive oil
- 1 ounce of kale, chopped
- 1 ounce of red onions, sliced
- 1 teaspoon chopped ginger

- 1.5 ounces of buckwheat

Directions:

1. It is best to prepare the salsa first: remove the stalk of the tomato, chop it finely and mix it well with the other ingredients.
2. Preheat the oven to 425 °. In the meantime, marinate the chicken breast in some olive oil and a teaspoon of turmeric.
3. Heat an ovenproof pan on the stove and sauté the marinated chicken for one minute on each side. Then bake in the oven for about 10 minutes, take out and cover with aluminum foil.
4. In the meantime, briefly steam the kale. In a small saucepan, heat the red onions and ginger with olive oil until they become translucent, then add the kale and heat again.
5. Prepare buckwheat according to package Directions, serve with meat and vegetables.

Nutrition:

- Calories: 104,
- Sodium: 33 mg,
- Dietary Fiber: 1.4 g,
- Total Fat: 4.1 g,
- Total Carbs: 16.3 g,
- Protein: 1.3 g.

4. Tofu With Cauliflower

Preparation time: 5 Minutes

Cooking time: 45 Minutes

Servings 2

Ingredients:

- 2 ounces of red pepper, seeded
- 1 Thai chilies, cut in two halves, seeded
- 2 cloves of garlic
- 1 teaspoon of olive oil
- 1 pinch of cumin
- 1 pinch of coriander
- Juice of a 1/4 lemon
- 7 ounces of tofu
- 7 ounces of cauliflower, roughly chopped
- 1 ounce of red onions, finely chopped
- 1 teaspoon finely chopped ginger
- 2 teaspoons turmeric
- 2-ounce dried tomatoes, finely chopped
- 2 ounces of parsley, chopped

Directions:

1. Preheat oven to 400 °. Slice the peppers and put them in an ovenproof dish with chili and garlic. Pour some olive oil over it, add the dried herbs, and put it in the oven until the peppers are soft about 20 minutes). Let it cool down, put the peppers together with the lemon juice in a blender and work it into a soft mass.
2. Cut the tofu in half and divide the halves into triangles. Place the tofu in a small casserole dish, cover with the paprika mixture and place in the oven for about 20 minutes.
3. Chop the cauliflower until the pieces are smaller than a grain of rice.

4. Then, in a small saucepan, heat the garlic, onions, chili and ginger with olive oil until they become transparent. Add turmeric and cauliflower, mix well and heat again. Remove from heat and add parsley and tomatoes, mix well. Serve with the tofu in the sauce.

Nutrition:

- Calories: 304,
- Sodium: 73 mg,
- Dietary Fiber: 1.4 g,
- Total Fat: 4.1 g,
- Total Carbs: 1.3 g,
- Protein: 0.3 g.

5. Horseradish Flaked Salmon Fillet & Kale

Preparation time: 10 minutes

Cooking time: 30 minutes

Servings: 1

- 7oz of skinless, boneless salmon fillet
- 1.5oz of green beans
- 1.7oz of kale
- 1 tablespoon extra-virgin olive oil
- ½ garlic clove, crushed
- 1.4oz red onion, chopped
- 1 tablespoon fresh chives, chopped
- 1 tablespoon freshly chopped flat-leaf parsley
- 1 tablespoon low fat *crème fraiche*
- 1tablespoon horseradish sauce
- Juice of ¼ lemon
- A pinch of salt and pepper

Direction:

1. Preheat the grill.
2. Sprinkle a salmon fillet with salt and pepper. Place under the grill for 10-15 minutes. Flake and set aside.
3. Using a steamer, cook the kale and green beans for 10 minutes.
4. In a skillet, warm the oil over a high heat. Add garlic and red onion and fry for 2-3 minutes. Toss in the kale and beans, and then cook for 1-2 minutes more.
5. Mix the chives, parsley, *crème fraiche*, horseradish, lemon juice, and flaked salmon.
6. Serve the kale and beans topped with the dressed flaked salmon.

Nutrition:

- Calories: 304,
- Sodium: 73 mg,

- Dietary Fiber: 1.4 g,
- Total Fat: 4.1 g,
- Total Carbs: 1.3 g,
- Protein: 0.3 g.

6. Indulgent Yogurt

Preparation Time: 10 minutes

Cooking Time: 0 minutes

Servings: 1

Ingredients:

- 125 mixed berries
- 3.5oz of Greek yogurt
- 25 walnuts, chopped
- 0.9oz of dark chocolate (at least 85% cocoa solids), grated

Directions:

1. Toss the mixed berries into a serving bowl. Cover with yogurt and top with chocolate and walnuts. Voila!

Nutrition:

- Calories:115
- Carbs: 4g
- Fat: 8g
- Protein: 6g

7. Frozen Gazpacho

Preparation time: 10 minutes

Cooking time: 0 minutes

Servings: 2

Ingredients:

- 2 large or 6 small tomatoes, chopped
- 1 avocado, seeded, sliced and picked (wait until prompted)
- 1 medium cucumber, chopped
- 1 small red onion, chopped
- 1 cup very finely chopped arugula
- ½ celery stalk, finely chopped
- 1 garlic clove, chopped or pressed
- ½ chili or a pinch of cayenne pepper
- 1 teaspoon of lime juice pinch of sea salt
- A pinch of pepper

Direction:

1. Put the ingredients in a blender or food processor and let them beat gently. You don't want to mix too well, or you make a liquid instead of a soup. The gazpacho must be thick. After mixing, put in the refrigerator for about 1 hour. You can also leave it overnight.
2. Cut and remove the avocado just before eating. Serve half of the gazpacho in a cold bowl. Add the avocado slices and serve immediately.

Nutrition:

- Calories: 304,
- Sodium: 73 mg,
- Dietary Fiber: 1.4 g,
- Total Fat: 4.1 g,
- Total Carbs: 1.3 g,
- Protein: 0.3 g.

8. Tomato Frittata

Preparation time: 10 minutes

Cooking time: 20 minutes

Servings: 2

Ingredients:

- 1.3oz cheddar cheese, grated
- 1.4oz kalamata olives, pitted and halved
- 8 cherry tomatoes, halved
- 4 large eggs
- 1 tablespoon fresh parsley, chopped
- 1 tablespoon fresh basil, chopped
- 1 tablespoon olive oil

Directions:

1. Whisk eggs together in a large mixing bowl. Toss in the parsley, basil, olives, tomatoes and cheese, stirring thoroughly.
2. In a small skillet, heat the olive oil over high heat. Pour in the frittata mixture and cook for 5-10 minutes, or set.
3. Remove the skillet from the hob and place under the grill for 5 minutes, or until firm and set. Divide into portions and serve immediately.

Nutrition:

- Calories: 304
- Sodium: 73 mg
- Dietary Fiber: 1.4 g
- Total Fat: 4.1 g
- Total Carbs: 1.3
- Protein: 0.3 g

9. Chicken With Kale and Chili Salsa

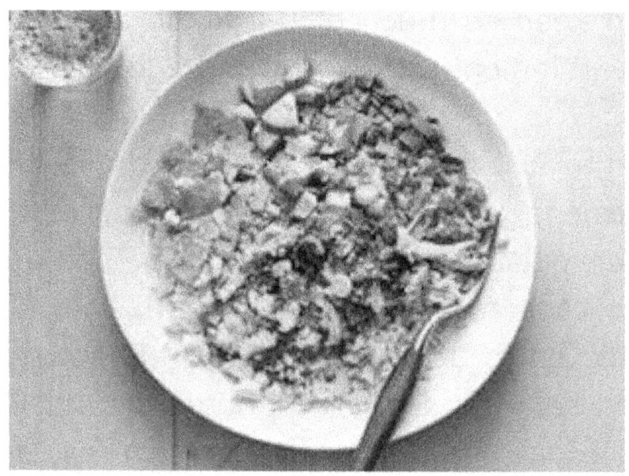

Preparation time: 5 Minutes

Cooking Time: 45 Minutes

Servings 1

Ingredients:

- 3 ounces of buckwheat
- 1 teaspoon of chopped fresh ginger
- Juice of ½ lemon, divided
- 2 teaspoons of ground turmeric
- 3 ounces of kale, chopped
- 1.3 ounces of red onion, sliced
- 4 ounces of skinless, boneless chicken breast
- 1 tablespoon of extra-virgin olive oil
- 1 tomato
- 1 handful parsley
- 1 bird's eye chili, chopped

Directions:

1. Start with the salsa: Remove the eye out of the tomato and finely chop it, making sure to keep as much of the liquid as you can. Mix it with the chili, parsley, and lemon juice. You could add everything to a blender for different results.
2. Heat your oven to 220 degrees F. Marinate the chicken with a little oil, 1 teaspoon of turmeric, and the lemon juice. Let it rest for 5-10 minutes.
3. Heat a pan over medium heat until it is hot, then add marinated chicken and allow it to cook for a minute on both sides until it is pale gold). Transfer the chicken to the oven if the pan is not ovenproof place it in a baking tray and bake for 8 to 10 minutes or until it is cooked through. Take the chicken out of the oven, cover with foil, and let it rest for five minutes before you serve.
4. Meanwhile, in a steamer, steam the kale for about 5 minutes.
5. In a little oil, fry the ginger and red onions until they are soft but not colored, and then add in the cooked kale and fry it for a minute.
6. Cook the buckwheat in accordance with the packet Directions with the remaining turmeric. Serve alongside the vegetables, salsa and chicken.

Nutrition:

- Calories: 304
- Sodium: 73 mg
- Dietary Fiber: 1.4 g
- Total Fat: 4.1 g
- Total Carbs: 1.3 g
- Protein: 0.3 g

10.   Buckwheat Tuna Casserole

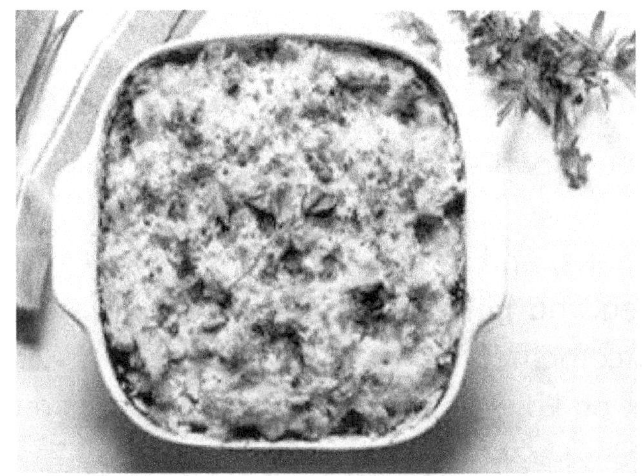

Preparation time: 10 minutes

Cooking time: 35 minutes

Servings: 2

Ingredients:

- 2 tablespoons butter
- 10-ounce package buckwheat ramen noodles
- 2 cups boiling water
- 1/3 cup dry red wine
- 3 cups milk
- 2 tablespoons dried parsley
- 2 teaspoons turmeric
- ½ teaspoon curry powder
- 2 tablespoons All-Purpose flour
- 2 cups celery, chopped
- 1 cup frozen peas
- 2 cans tuna, drained

Directions:

1. Dot butter into your crockpot and grease the pot.
2. Place buckwheat ramen noodles in a large bowl and pour boiling water to cover. Let sit for 5 – 8 minutes, or until noodles separate when prodded with a fork.
3. In a separate bowl, whisk together red wine, milk, parsley, turmeric and flour.
4. Fold in celery, peas, and tuna.
5. Drain the ramen and place into crockpot, pouring the tuna mixture over the top. Mix to combine.
6. Cover and cook on Low 7 to 9 hours, stirring occasionally.

Nutrition:

- Calories: 304
- Sodium: 73 mg
- Dietary Fiber: 1.4 g
- Total Fat: 4.1 g
- Total Carbs: 1.3 g
- Protein: 0.3 g

11.   Cheesy Crockpot Chicken andVegetables

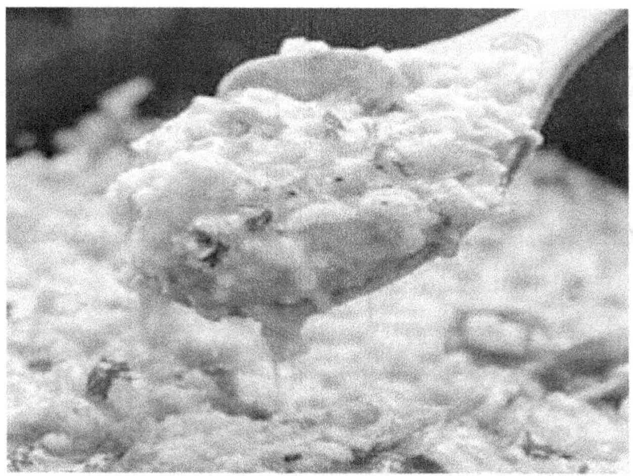

Preparation time: 10 minutes

Cooking time: 45 minutes

Servings: 2

Ingredients:

- 1/3 cup ham, diced
- 3 carrots, chopped
- 3 stalks celery, chopped
- 1 small yellow onion, diced
- 2 cups mushrooms, sliced
- 1 cup green beans, chopped
- ¼ cup water
- 4 boneless, skinless chicken breasts, cubed
- 1 cup chicken broth
- 1 cup milk
- 1 tablespoon parsley, chopped
- ¾ teaspoon poultry seasoning
- 1 tablespoon All-Purpose flour

- 1 cup cheddar cheese, shredded
- ¼ cup Parmesan, shredded

Directions:

1. In a large bowl, combine ham, carrots, celery, onion, mushrooms, and green beans. Mix and transfer to your crockpot.
2. Layer the chicken on top, without mixing.
3. In the bowl, now empty, whisk broth, milk, parsley, poultry seasoning and flour together until well combined.
4. Fold in the cheddar and Parmesan.
5. Pour the mixture over the chicken. DO NOT STIR.
6. Cover and cook on high 3-4 hours, or low 6-8 hours.

Nutrition:

- Calories: 314
- Sodium: 73 mg
- Dietary Fiber: 2.4 g
- Total Fat: 5.1 g
- Total Carbs: 1.3g
- Protein: 5.3 g

12.   Artichoke, Chicken and Capers

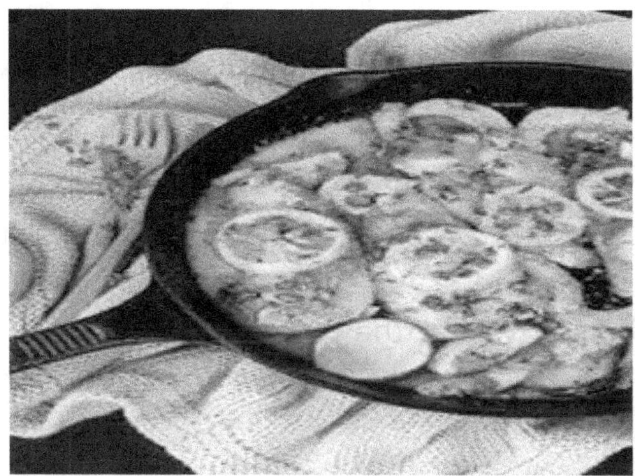

Preparation time: 10 minutes

Cooking time: 55 minutes

Servings: 2

Ingredients:

- 6 boneless, skinless chicken breasts
- 2 cups mushrooms, sliced
- 1 (14 ½ ounces) can diced tomatoes
- 1 (8 or 9 ounces) package frozen artichokes
- 1 cup chicken broth
- ¼ cup dry white wine
- 1 medium yellow onion, diced
- ½ cup Kalamata olives, sliced
- ¼ cup capers, drained
- 3 tablespoons chia seeds
- 3 teaspoons curry powder
- 1 teaspoon turmeric
- 3/4 teaspoon dried lovage

- Salt and pepper to taste
- 3 cups hot cooked buckwheat

Directions:

1. Rinse chicken & set aside.
2. In a large bowl, combine mushrooms, tomatoes – with juice, frozen artichoke hearts, chicken broth, white wine, onion, olives and capers.
3. Stir in chia seeds, curry powder, turmeric, lovage, salt and pepper.
4. Pour half the mixture into your crockpot, add the chicken, and pour the remainder of the sauce over the top.
5. Cover and cook on Low for 7 to 8 hours or on High for 3 1/2 to 4 hours.
6. Serve with hot cooked buckwheat.

Nutrition:

- Calories: 314,
- Sodium: 73 mg,
- Dietary Fiber: 2.4 g,
- Total Fat: 5.1 g,
- Total Carbs: 1.3 g,
- Protein: 5.3 g.

13.   Chicken Merlot With Mushrooms

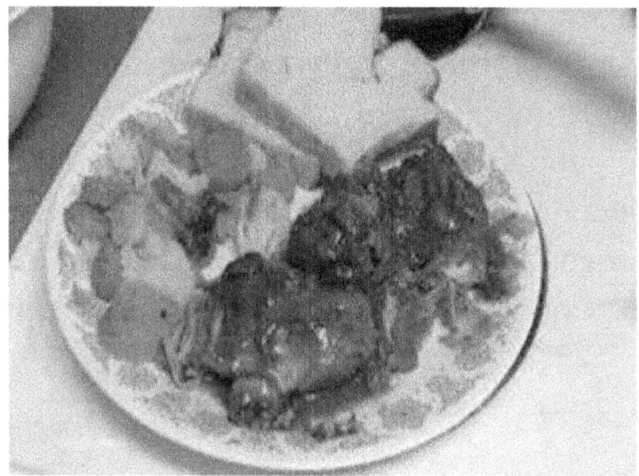

Preparation time: 10 minutes

Cooking time: 40 minutes

Servings: 2

Ingredients:

- 6 boneless, skinless chicken breasts, cubed
- 3 cups mushrooms, sliced
- 1 large red onion, chopped
- 2 cloves garlic, minced
- ¾ cup chicken broth
- 1 (6 ounces) can tomato paste
- ¼ cup Merlot
- 3 tablespoons chia seeds
- 2 tablespoons basil, chopped finely
- 2 teaspoons sugar
- Salt and pepper to taste
- 1 (10 ounces) package buckwheat ramen noodles, cooked
- 2 tablespoons Parmesan, shaved

Directions:

1. Rinse chicken; set aside.
2. Add mushrooms, onion, and garlic to the crockpot and mix.
3. Place chicken cubes on top of the vegetables and do not mix.
4. In a large bowl, combine broth, tomato paste, wine, chia seeds, basil, sugar, salt, and pepper. Pour over the chicken.
5. Cover and cook on low for 7 to 8 hours or on high for 3 ½ to 4 hours.
6. To serve, spoon chicken, mushroom mixture, and sauce over hot cooked buckwheat ramen noodles. Top with shaved Parmesan.

Nutrition:

- Calories: 314,
- Sodium: 73 mg,
- Dietary Fiber: 2.4 g,
- Total Fat: 5.1 g,
- Total Carbs: 1.3 g,
- Protein: 5.3 g.

14. Country Chicken Breasts

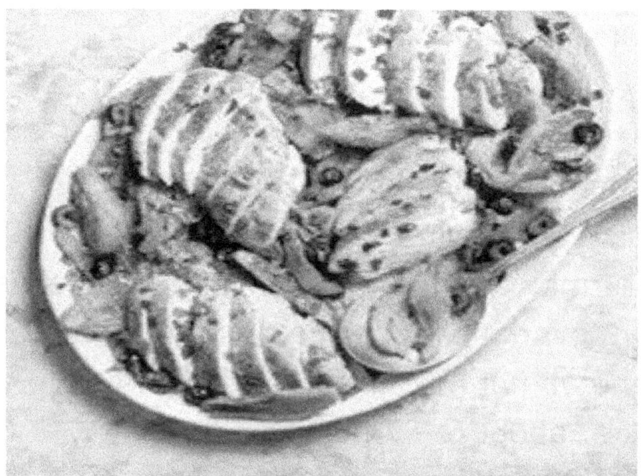

Preparation time: 10 minutes

Cooking time: 45 minutes

Servings: 2

Ingredients:

- 2 medium green apples, diced
- 1 small red onion, finely diced
- 1 small green bell pepper, chopped
- 3 cloves garlic, minced
- 2 tablespoons dried currants
- 1 tablespoon curry powder
- 1 teaspoon turmeric
- 1 teaspoon ground ginger
- ¼ teaspoon chili pepper flakes
- 1 can (14 ½ ounce) diced tomatoes
- 6 skinless, boneless chicken breasts, halved
- ½ cup chicken broth
- 1 cup long-grain white rice

- 1-pound large raw shrimp, shelled and deveined
- Salt and pepper to taste
- Chopped parsley
- 1/3 cup slivered almonds

Directions

1. Rinse chicken, pat dry, and set aside.
2. In a large crockpot, combine apples, onion, bell pepper, garlic, currants, curry powder, turmeric, ginger, and chili pepper flakes. Stir in tomatoes.
3. Arrange chicken, overlapping pieces slightly, on top of tomato mixture.
4. Pour in broth and do not mix or stir.
5. Cover and cook at about 6 – 7 hours on low.
6. Preheat oven to 200 degrees F.
7. Carefully transfer chicken to an oven-safe plate, cover lightly, and keep warm in the oven.
8. Stir rice into the remaining liquid. Increase cooker heat setting to high; cover and cook, stirring once or twice, until rice is almost tender to bite, 30 to 35 minutes. Stir in shrimp, cover, and cook until shrimp are opaque in center, about 10 more minutes.
9. Meanwhile, toast almonds in a small pan over medium heat until golden brown, 5 - 8 minutes, stirring occasionally. Set aside.
10. To serve, season rice mixture to taste with salt and pepper. Mound in a warm serving dish and arrange chicken on top. Sprinkle with parsley and almonds.

Nutrition:

- Calories: 314,
- Sodium: 73 mg,
- Dietary Fiber: 2.4 g,
- Total Fat: 5.1 g,
- Total Carbs: 1.3 g,
- Protein: 5.3 g.

15.   Tuna and Kale

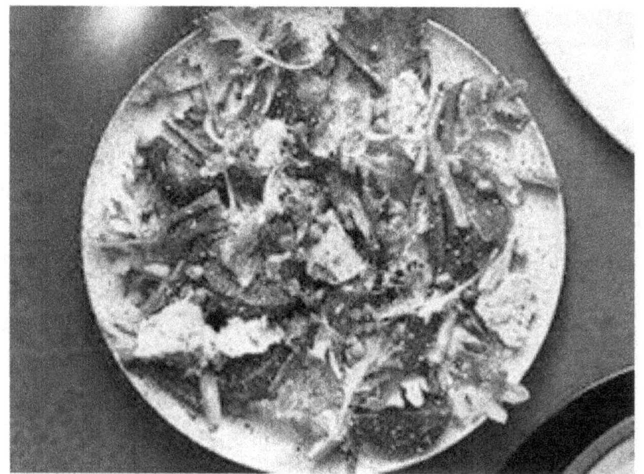

Preparation time: 5 minutes

Cooking time: 20 minutes

Servings: 4

Ingredients:

- 1-pound tuna fillets, boneless, skinless and cubed
- 2 tablespoons olive oil
- 1 cup kale, torn
- ½ cup cherry tomatoes, cubed
- 1 yellow onion, chopped

Directions:

1. Heat up a pan with the oil over medium heat, add the onion and sauté for 5 minutes.
2. Add the tuna and the other ingredients, toss, cook everything for 15 minutes more, divide between plates and serve.

Nutrition:

- Calories: 314,
- Sodium: 73 mg,
- Dietary Fiber: 2.4 g,

- Total Fat: 5.1 g,
- Total Carbs: 1.3 g,
- Protein: 5.3 g.

16.   Turkey With Cauliflower Couscous

Preparation time: 20 minutes

Cooking time: 50 minutes

Servings: 1

Ingredients:

- 3 ounces of turkey
- 2-ounce g of cauliflower
- 2 ounces of red onion
- 1 teaspoon fresh ginger
- 1 pepper Bird's Eye
- 1 clove of garlic
- 3 tablespoons of extra virgin olive oil
- 2 teaspoons of turmeric
- 1.3 ounces of dried tomatoes
- 0.3ounces parsley
- Dried sage to taste
- 1 tablespoon of capers
- 1/4 of fresh lemon juice

Directions:

1. Blend the raw cauliflower tops and cook them in a teaspoon of extra virgin olive oil, garlic, red onion, chili pepper, ginger, and a teaspoon of turmeric.
2. Leave to flavor on the fire for a minute, then add the chopped sun-dried tomatoes and 5 g of parsley. Season the turkey slice with a teaspoon of extra virgin olive oil, the dried sage and cook it in another teaspoon of extra virgin olive oil. Once ready, season with a tablespoon of capers, 1/4 of lemon juice, 5 g of parsley, a tablespoon of water and add the cauliflower.

Nutrition:

- Calories: 114,
- Sodium: 7.3 mg,
- Dietary Fiber: 2.4 g,
- Total Fat: 2.1 g,
- Total Carbs: 1.3 g,
- Protein: 5.3 g.

17.　Oriental Prawns With Buckwheat

Preparation time: 20 minutes

Cooking time: 20 minutes

Servings: 1

Ingredients:

- 3 ounces of shrimps
- 1 spoon of turmeric
- 1 spoon of extra-virgin oil
- 1.3 ounces of grain spaghetti
- Cooking water
- Salt
- 1 clove of garlic
- Bird's Eye chili
- 1 spoon of ginger
- Red onion
- 3 ounces of celery
- 1.3 ounces of green beans
- 1.7 ounces of kale
- Broth

Directions:

1. Cook for 2-3 minutes the peeled prawns with 1 teaspoon of turmeric and 1 teaspoon of extra virgin olive oil. Boil the buckwheat noodles in salt-free water, drain and set aside.
2. Fry with another teaspoon of extra virgin olive oil, 1 clove of garlic, 1 Bird's Eye chili and 1 teaspoon of finely chopped fresh ginger, 20 g of red onion and 40 g of sliced celery, 75 g of chopped green beans, 50 g of curly kale roughly chopped.
3. Add 100 ml of broth and bring to a boil, letting it simmer until the vegetables are cooked and soft. Add the prawns, spaghetti, and 5 g of celery leaves, bring to the boil, and serve.

Nutrition:

- Calories: 114,
- Sodium: 7.3 mg,
- Dietary Fiber: 2.4 g,
- Total Fat: 2.1 g,
- Total Carbs: 1.3 g,
- Protein: 5.3 g.

18.   Miso and Tofu With Sesame Glaze and Sautéed Vegetables in a Pan With Ginger and Chili

Preparation time: 20 minutes

Cooking time: 10 minutes

Servings: 1

Ingredients:

- 2 teaspoons of extra virgin olive oil
- 7 ounces of mushrooms (enoki or champignon)
- ½ carrot, peeled and cut into julienne strips
- 1 red chili peppers, sliced
- 1 tablespoon of fresh ginger
- Cabbage or spinach
- Onion
- Miso paste
- 125 g of tofu

Directions:

1. Heat the oil in a large pan and add the mushrooms and carrot. Quickly cook the vegetables for 1minute or as long as they are tender, add the chili, the ginger and cook for 10 seconds.
2. Add the cabbage or spinach and ì onions in the pan and cook until the leaves are slightly wilted. Remove them from the pans and divide them into two bowls.
3. Bring 700 ml of water to the boiling point in a large saucepan. In a small bowl, mix the miso with a couple of teaspoons of water and add it to the pot. Stir to mix and still incorporate miso if necessary. Divide the drained and diced tofu into the bowls and cover with the miso broth. Add tamari or soy sauce and serve immediately.

Nutrition:

- Calories: 114,

- Sodium: 7.3 mg,
- Dietary Fiber: 2.4 g,
- Total Fat: 2.1 g,
- Total Carbs: 1.3 g,
- Protein: 5.3 g.

19.   Blueberry Banana Pancakes

Preparation time: 10 minutes

Cooking time: 10 minutes

Servings: 1

Ingredients:

- 3 bananas
- 3 eggs
- 75 g rolled oats
- A pinch of salt
- 1 teaspoon baking powder
- ¾ cup of blueberries (fresh or frozen)

Directions:

1. To complete this recipe, you will need to do the following:
2. Put your oats into a blender or food processor and pulse until you have created an oat flour.
3. In your blender or food processor, add in everything but the blueberries. Pulse it together for roughly 2 minutes until it is well combined and you have a nice, smooth batter.
4. Pour the batter into a large mixing bowl and gently add in the blueberries, folding them in rather than mixing it up. Make sure that you do not overmix.
5. Wait 10 minutes, allowing the baking powder to activate.
6. Heat a frying pan to medium-high and add a small amount of oil or butter to the surface so that the pancake does not stick. Scoop in the blueberry banana batter to the size desired and allowed it to fry until the bottom is golden brown and ready to flip.
7. Flip and cook the other side until also golden brown.

Nutrition:

- Calories: 495

- Sodium: 32 mg
- Dietary Fiber: 1.4 g
- Total Fat: 2.6 g
- Total Carbs: 12.3 g
- Protein: 1.3 g

20.   Breakfast Chocolate Muffins

Preparation time: 10 minutes

Cooking time: 30 minutes

Servings: 1

Ingredients:

- Almond paste
- Banana (Blackberry)
- 1 Egg
- 1 Teaspoon vanilla extract
- 1/2 teaspoon tartar yeast
- 100 grams of chocolate chips

Directions:

1. Preheat the oven to 200 ° C and prepare a baking tray made of paper or silicone muffins.
2. Put all ingredients (except optional chocolate chips) in a food processor and mix it in a smooth, sticky dough.
3. Optional: add and mix chocolate bars
4. Optional: add and incorporate chocolate bars
5. Place the dough in a muffin pan and bake until golden, then cook for about 12-15 minutes.

Nutrition:

- Calories: 205
- Sodium: 32 mg
- Dietary Fiber: 1.5 g
- Total Fat: 5.1 g
- Total Carbs: 16.4 g
- Protein: 1.3 g

21.   Cauliflower Couscous

Preparation time: 20 minutes

Cooking time: 10 minutes

Servings: 1

Ingredients:

- 28-ounces cauliflower
- 7 dried tomatoes
- 1 tablespoon of capers
- 1 anchovy in oil
- 2 tablespoons of pitted Taggiasca olives
- 1 clove of garlic
- 7 ounces of marinated anchovies
- Fresh oregano
- Extra virgin olive oil

Directions:

1. To prepare the cauliflower couscous, remove the leaves and remove the florets. Rinse the couscous under running freshwater, dab them with kitchen paper to dry them and blend them, a little at a time, in a food processor and transfer the granules obtained in a clean bowl.
2. Let the dried tomatoes soak in lukewarm water for half an hour, then squeeze them, dab them with paper towels and cut them into thin strips. Drain the capers and chop half of them with a knife. Coarsely chop also half of the olives. Peel the garlic and mash it with the palm of your hand. In a large pan, heat a little oil. Fry the garlic with the capers (chopped and whole), the anchovy, and the chopped olives. Also, add the sliced tomatoes over high heat.
3. Pour the cauliflower grains and stir in with a little water (about half a glass: the cauliflower must remain crunchy), always on high heat, and stir. Add salt, turn off the heat and add the anchovies marinated in fillets, the remaining olives, a little fresh oregano leaves and a round of raw oil.

4. Serve the cauliflower couscous, hot or cold, depending on your taste.

Nutrition:

- Calories: 114,
- Sodium: 7.3 mg,
- Dietary Fiber: 2.4 g,
- Total Fat: 2.1 g,
- Total Carbs: 1.3 g,
- Protein: 5.3 g.

22.   Turkey Escalopes With Sage, Parsley, and Capers

Preparation time: 20 minutes

Cooking time: 10 minutes

Servings: 1

Ingredients:

- 8 slices of turkey
- Half white onion
- 1 large sprig of parsley
- A few fresh sage leaves or a nice pinch of the dried one
- Olive oil to taste
- Salt
- Capers
- Flour

Directions:

1. Cover the turkey slices with flour once at the time, shake them slightly to remove excess flour. Wash parsley, sage, and finely chop them with a knife, add the capers. Finely chop the onion, heat up 2 tablespoons of oil in a pan, add the onion, fry 1 minute, add 2 tablespoons of water, lower the heat, cover and cook the onion, add 3 tablespoons of oil, raise the heat, put on the heat the slices of turkey in the pan, brown them on both sides, salt.
2. One minute before turning off the heat, sprinkle the slices with the chopped sage and parsley with capers. Serve with the sauce made from the pan.

Nutrition:

- Calories: 120,
- Sodium: 23 mg,
- Dietary Fiber: 2.4 g,
- Total Fat: 2.1 g,

- Total Carbs: 1.3 g,
- Protein: 10.3 g.

23.   Cabbage and Red Onion Dahl With Buckwheat

Preparation time: 20 minutes

Cooking time: 30 minutes

Servings: 1

Ingredients:

- 7.5-ounces hulled buckwheat
- 1.5ounces of curly cabbage
- Vegetable broth
- 1 Tomato pulp
- 2 spoons of extra virgin olive oil
- Red onion
- Basil
- Chopped chili pepper
- Water
- Pepper
- Salt

Directions:

1. Pour the water into a pot, add the oil and, to the fire, wait until it boils and add the broth. Then turn off the heat. Meanwhile, wash the cauliflower, cut the florets into small pieces and drain them. Chop the shallot finely enough. Pour the buckwheat in a colander and rinse it under running water.

2. In another saucepan (large) pour two full spoons of oil, add the chopped shallot, the mince for sautéing and fry it on a soft flame, often mixing to prevent it from sticking to the pot. When the onion is transparent and dried, add the buckwheat and toast it for a few minutes, mixing without letting it stick to the bottom of the pot. Then add the tomato pulp, broth, chopped basil, chopped red pepper, and mix, then add the cauliflower florets.

3. Cook the Buckwheat and cauliflower soup for 30 minutes, covering the pan with a lid and on low heat, occasionally stirring so as not to stick the buckwheat to the pan. If necessary, season with salt. After cooking, serve the buckwheat and cauliflower soup with freshly ground pepper. If you like (and if you are not vegan, vegetarian or lactose intolerant), you could also add some grated pecorino cheese. Your buckwheat and cauliflower soup is ready!

Nutrition:

- Calories: 120,
- Sodium: 23 mg,
- Dietary Fiber: 2.4 g,
- Total Fat: 2.1 g,
- Total Carbs: 1.3 g,
- Protein: 10.3 g.

24.   Mushroom and Tofu Scramble

Preparation time: 10 minutes

Cooking time: 20 minutes

Servings: 2

Ingredients:

- 7 ounces of extra firm tofu
- 2 teaspoon turmeric powder
- 1 teaspoon black pepper
- 1.5ounces of kale, roughly chopped
- 2 teaspoon extra virgin olive oil
- 1.5 ounces of red onion, thinly sliced
- 1 Thai chilies, thinly sliced
- 100g mushrooms, thinly sliced
- 4 tablespoons parsley, finely chopped

Directions:

1. Wrap the tofu in paper towels and place something heavy on top to help it drain.
2. Mix the turmeric with a little water until you achieve a light paste.
3. Steam the kale for 2 to 3 minutes.
4. Heat the olive oil in a frying pan over medium heat until hot but not smoking, add the onion, chili, and mushrooms and fry for 2 to 3 minutes until they have started to brown and soften.
5. Crumble the tofu into bite-size pieces and add to the pan, pour the turmeric paste over the tofu, and mix thoroughly. Add the black pepper and stir. Cook over medium heat for 2 to 3 minutes, so the spices are cooked through and the tofu has started to brown.
6. Add the kale and continue to cook over medium heat for another minute. Finally, add the parsley, mix well, and serve.

Nutrition:

- Calories: 123
- Sodium: 36 mg
- Dietary Fiber: 2.4 g
- Total Fat: 4.7 g
- Total Carbs: 16.3 g
- Protein: 1.3 g

25.   Kale Scramble

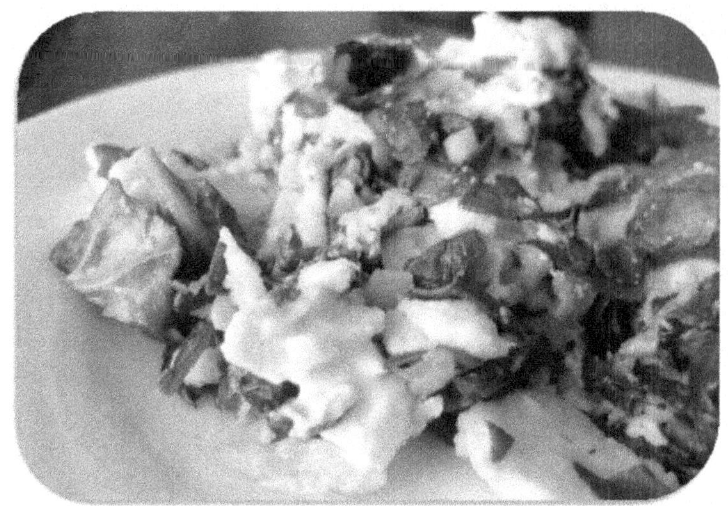

Preparation time: 10 minutes

Cooking time: 6 minutes

Total time: 16 minutes

Servings: 2

Ingredients:

- 4 eggs
- 1/8 teaspoon ground turmeric
- Salt and ground black pepper, to taste
- 1 tablespoon water
- 2 teaspoons olive oil
- 1 cup fresh kale, tough ribs removed and chopped

Directions:

1. In a bowl, add the eggs, turmeric, salt, black pepper, and water and with a whisk, beat until foamy.
2. In a wok, heat the oil over medium heat.

3. Add the egg mixture and stir to combine.
4. Immediately, reduce the heat to medium-low and cook for about 1–2 minutes, stirring frequently.
5. Stir in the kale and cook for about 3–4 minutes, stirring frequently.
6. Remove from the heat and serve immediately.

Nutrition:

- Calories: 183
- Sodium: 35 mg
- Dietary Fiber: 2.4 g
- Total Fat: 4.1 g
- Total Carbs: 16.8 g
- Protein: 1.6 g

26.   Apple Pancakes With Blackcurrant Compote

Preparation time: 10 minutes

Cooking time: 20 minutes

Servings: 2

Ingredients:

- 4 ounces of porridge oats
- 1.8 ounces of plain flour
- 1 tablespoon caster sugar
- ½ teaspoon baking powder
- 1 large green apple, peeled, cored and cut into small pieces
- 150ml semi-skimmed milk
- I large egg white
- 1 teaspoon light olive oil

For the compote:

- 1.5 ounces of blackcurrants washed and stalks removed.
- 1 tablespoon caster sugar
- 2 tablespoons water

Directions:

1. Make the compote first. Place the blackcurrants, sugar, and water in a small pan. Bring to a simmer and cook for 10-15 minutes.
2. Place the Oats, flour, baking powder, and caster sugar in a large bowl and mix properly.
3. Stir the apple into the powder mixture and then whisk in the milk a little at a time until you have a smooth mixture.
4. Whisk the egg white to a stiff peak and then fold into the pancake batter.
5. Heat ½ teaspoon olive oil in a non-stick frying pan on medium heat and pour ½ of the batter. Reduce heat and allow the pancake to cook properly, flip to the other side with a spatula. Cook both sides until golden brown. Remove and repeat to make 2 pancakes.

6. Serve the pancakes with the blackcurrant compote drizzled over.

Nutrition:

- 123 calories

27.   Mushroom Scramble Egg

Preparation Time: 5 minutes

Cooking Time: 10 minutes

Servings: 3

Ingredients:

- Two eggs
- 1 teaspoon ground turmeric
- 1 teaspoon mild curry powder
- 20g kale, roughly chopped
- 1 teaspoon extra virgin olive oil
- ½ bird's eye chili, thinly sliced
- A handful of thinly sliced, button mushrooms
- 5g parsley, finely chopped

Directions:

1. Mix the curry and turmeric powder, then add a little water until a light paste has been achieved.
2. Steam up the kale 2–3 minutes.
3. On medium heat, heat the oil in a frying pan and fry the chili and mushrooms for 2–3 minutes till they start browning and softening.
4. Put the eggs and spice paste, and cook over medium heat, then add the kale and start cooking for another minute over medium heat. Add the parsley, then mix well and serve.

Nutrition:

- Calories: 182,
- Sodium: 23 mg,
- Dietary Fiber: 1.5 g,
- Total Fat: 3.1 g,
- Total Carbs: 14.3 g,
- Protein: 2.3 g.

28.   Sirtfood Mushroom Scramble Eggs

Preparation time: 10 minutes

Cooking time: 20 minutes

Servings: 1

Ingredients:

- 2 medium eggs
- I teaspoon turmeric
- 1 ounce of kale, roughly chopped
- 1 teaspoon extra virgin olive oil
- 1/2 chili, thinly sliced
- 0.5 ounces of red onions
- Parsley, thinly chopped
- A handful of button mushrooms, thinly sliced

Directions:

1. Steam the kale for 2-3 minutes.
2. Mix the turmeric powder with water to form a light paste.
3. Break into a bowl and whisk, add the turmeric paste, parsley, and mix properly.
4. Heat the olive oil in a non-stick frying pan over medium heat and fry the onion, chili, and mushroom until they have started to brown and soften.
5. Add the steamed kale to the mixture in the frying pan and stir.
6. Pour the egg mixture into the frying pan and stir.
7. Reduce the heat and allow the egg to cook and stir.

Nutrition:

- Calories: 104
- Sodium: 27 mg
- Dietary Fiber: 2.4 g
- Total Fat: 2.1 g
- Total Carbs: 13.3 g
- Protein: 1.8 g

29.   Aromatic Chicken Breast With Kale, Red Onion, Tomato Sauce And Chili

Preparation time: 20 minutes

Cooking time: 50 minutes

Servings: 1

Ingredients:

- 1 teaspoon aromatic herbs
- Chili pepper
- Aromatic chicken breast
- Cabbage
- Red onion
- Tomato sauce

Directions:

1. Boil the chicken. Peel, stick and wash the carrot. Wash the celery stick, then peel and wash the shallot. Cut the vegetables into chunks. Bring 2 liters of water to a boil with cabbage, red onion and tomato sauce. Simmer the broth for about 15 minutes. Soak the chicken breast for about 25 minutes in the aromatic broth. Turn off the heat and let it cool in the cooking liquid.
2. Arrange the chicken breast on a cutting board, remove the central bone and cartilage. Cut the 2 halves with a sharp knife into 1 cm thick slices. Put a few grains of pink pepper between two sheets of parchment paper and chop them with the meat mallet.
3. Divide the slices into individual plates and garnish each plate.
4. Serve with the sauce.

Nutrition:

- Calories: 120,
- Sodium: 23 mg,
- Dietary Fiber: 2.4 g,
- Total Fat: 2.1 g,

- Total Carbs: 1.3 g,
- Protein: 10.3 g.

30.   Buckwheat With Mushrooms and Green Onions

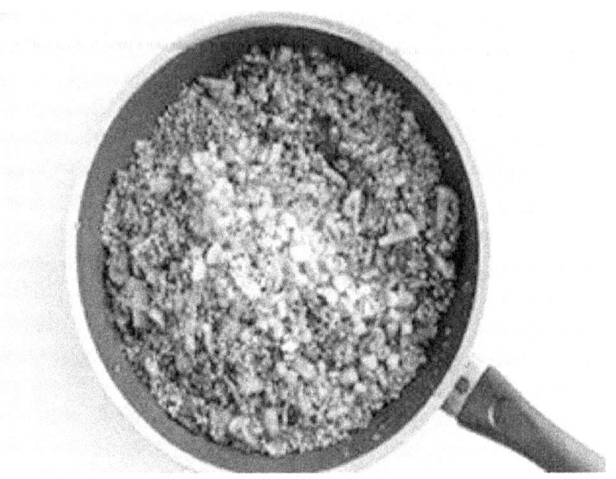

Preparation time: 10 minutes

Cooking time: 40 minutes

Servings: 2

Ingredients:

- 1 cup buckwheat groats
- 2 cups vegetable or chicken broth
- 3 green onions, thinly sliced
- 1 cup mushrooms, sliced
- Salt and pepper to taste
- 2 teaspoons butter

Directions:

1. Combine all ingredients in your crockpot. Cover and cook on low for 4 to 4 1/2 hours.

Nutrition:

- Calorie: 341
- Sodium: 38 mg
- Dietary Fiber: 1.4 g

- Total Fat: 3.1 g
- Total Carbs: 14.3 g
- Protein: 1.6 g

31.   Apples and Cabbage Mix

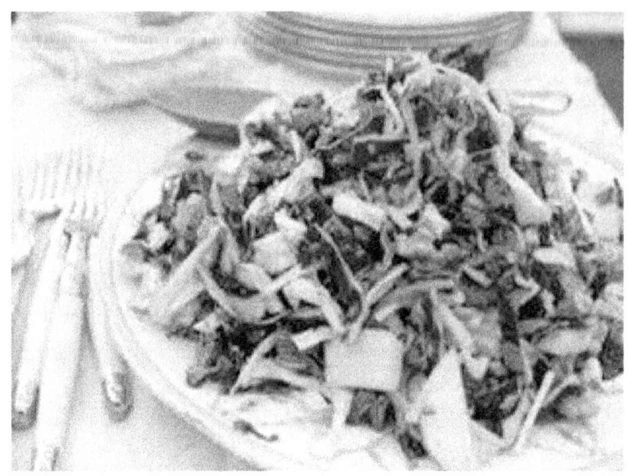

Preparation time: 5 minutes

Cooking time: 0 minute

Servings: 4

Ingredients:

- 2 cored and cubed green apples
- 2 tablespoons balsamic vinegar
- ½ teaspoon of caraway seeds
- 2 tablespoons of olive oil
- Black pepper
- 1 shredded red cabbage head

Directions:

1. In a bowl, combine the cabbage with the apples and the other ingredients, toss and serve.

Nutrition:

- Calories: 165
- Sodium: 34 mg
- Dietary Fiber: 1.6 g

- Total Fat: 4.5 g
- Total Carbs: 16.5 g
- Protein: 1.4 g

32.   Moroccan Chicken Casserole

Preparation Time: 10 minutes

Cooking Time: 15 minutes

Servings: 4

Ingredients:

- 9 ounces of tinned chickpeas garbanzo beans drained
- 4 chicken breasts, cubed
- 4 Medrol dates, halved
- 6 dried apricots, halved
- 1 red onion, sliced
- 1 carrot, chopped
- 1 teaspoon ground cumin
- 1 teaspoon ground cinnamon
- 1 teaspoon ground turmeric
- 1 bird's-eye chili, chopped
- 1 pint's chicken stock broth
- 1 ounce of corn flour
- 2fl oz. water
- 2 tablespoons fresh coriander

Directions:

1. Place the chicken, chickpeas garbanzo beans, onion, carrot, chili, cumin, turmeric, cinnamon and stock broth into a large saucepan.
2. Put it to the boil, and reduce heat after that simmer for 25 minutes. Add in the dates and apricots and simmer for 10 minutes.
3. In a cup, mix the corn flour together with the water until it becomes a smooth paste. Pour the mixture into the saucepan and stir until it thickens. Add in the coriander cilantro and mix well. Serve with buckwheat or couscous.

Nutrition:

- Calories: 254
- Sodium: 32 mg
- Dietary Fiber: 1.7 g
- Total Fat: 4.1 g
- Total Carbs: 16.3 g
- Protein: 1.5 g

33.   Serrano Ham & Rocket Arugula

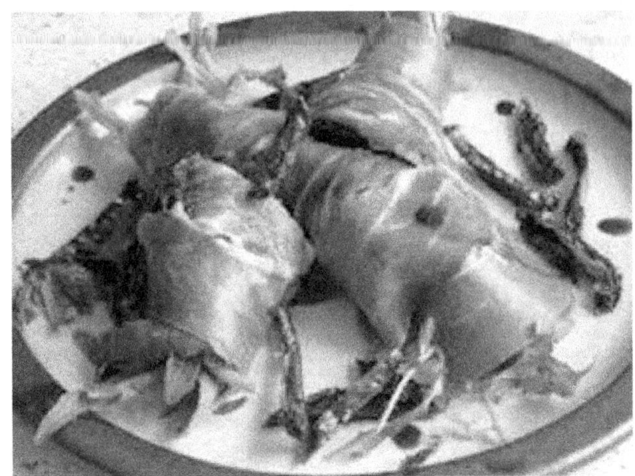

Preparation time: 5 Minutes

Cooking Time: 60 Minutes

Servings 2

Ingredients:

- 6 ounces of Serrano ham
- 4 ounces of rocket arugula leaves
- 2 tablespoons olive oil
- 1 tablespoon orange juice

Directions:

1. Pour the oil and juice into a bowl and toss the rocket arugula in the mixture. Serve the rocket onto plates and top it off with the ham.

Nutrition:

- Calories per serving: 165.3
- Sodium: 33 mg
- Dietary Fiber: 1.2 g
- Total Fat: 4.3 g

- Total Carbs: 16.3 g
- Protein: 1.6 g

34.   Strawberry Chocolate Chip Buckwheat Pancakes

Preparation time: 10 minutes

Cooking time: 20 minutes

Servings: 1

Ingredients:

- 1 cup of buckwheat flour
- 2 tablespoon coconut sugar or honey
- 1 teaspoon baking powder
- 1 teaspoon cinnamon powder
- ¼ teaspoon salt
- ¾ cup of soy milk
- 2 tablespoon olive oil (for cooking)
- 1 egg
- ½ cup finely chopped strawberries
- ¼ cup 85% dark chocolate, chopped finely (chips work as well)
- Any toppings you want

Directions:

1. To complete this recipe, you will need to do the following:
2. Grease your skillet lightly and preheat it at medium heat
3. Mix your dry ingredients together, holding the chocolate chips and strawberries.
4. Mix your wet ingredients together in a separate bowl, still holding the chocolate chips and strawberries
5. Mix in the strawberries and chocolate chips gently, folding them. Do not overmix
6. Using ½ cup of batter per pancake, add your first scoop to the skillet—you should get one that is roughly 5 inches wide

7. Cook for 5 minutes, or until the edges are cooking and it is bubbling on top. Flip, then cook another 2 minutes.
8. Repeat, lightly greasing your pan between pancakes you should have four pancakes.

Nutrition:

- Calories: 495
- Sodium: 33 mg
- Dietary Fiber: 1.4 g
- Total Fat: 4.1 g
- Total Carbs: 16.7 g
- Protein: 1.3 g

35.   Spiced Scrambled Eggs

Preparation time: 10 minutes

Cooking time: 20 minutes

Servings: 2

Ingredients:

- 2 teaspoon extra virgin olive oil
- 1/4 cup (40g) red onion, finely chopped
- 1/2 bell pepper, finely chopped
- 6 medium eggs
- 1/2 cup (100ml) milk
- 1 teaspoon ground turmeric
- 4 tablespoons (10g) parsley, finely chopped

Directions:

1. Heat the oil in a frying pan and fry the red onion and bell pepper until soft but not browned.
2. Whisk the eggs, milk, turmeric, and parsley. Add to the hot pan and continue cooking over low to medium heat, constantly moving the egg mixture around the pan to scramble it and stop it from sticking/burning.
3. When you have achieved your desired consistency, serve

Nutrition:

- Calories: 235
- Sodium: 32 mg
- Dietary Fiber: 2.4 g
- Total Fat: 4.2 g
- Total Carbs: 16.2 g

36.   Baked Tofu With Harissa

Preparation time: 20 minutes

Cooking time: 50 minutes

Servings: 1

Ingredients:

- Tofu
- Cherry tomatoes
- Capers in salt
- Oregano
- Extra virgin olive oil
- Fresh chili
- Garlic 4 cloves
- Fresh coriander in leaves 1 tablespoon
- Coriander powder 1 tablespoon
- Dried mint 1 tablespoon
- Extra virgin olive oil to taste
- Salt up to 1 tablespoon
- Caraway seeds 1 tablespoon

Directions:

1. Cut the tofu into slices of 100gr each, cut the cherry tomatoes in half. Place each slice of tofu in the center of a 20x20cm large sheet of parchment paper and season it with cherry tomatoes, capers, olives, oregano, and evo oil. Close the toffee paper and bake at 250 ° C for 15min.
2. To prepare the Harissa, remove the stalks from the chilies, wash them, cut them, remove the internal seeds, and leave them to soak in a little water for at least 1 hour.
3. After the hour, drain and crush them together with the other ingredients, or put everything in a mixer, and add as much oil as needed to make a very thick cream.

4. Put the mixture in a glass jar and cover the surface with oil, which will serve to preserve the Harissa.

Nutrition:

- Calories: 120,
- Sodium: 23 mg,
- Dietary Fiber: 2.4 g,
- Total Fat: 2.1 g,
- Total Carbs: 1.3 g,
- Protein: 10.3 g.

37. Pan-Fried Salmon Fillet With Caramelized Radicchio Salad, Rocket and Celery Leaves

Preparation time: 20 minutes

Cooking time: 30 minutes

Servings: 1

Ingredients:

- Salmon Slices
- 8 oranges
- 1 lemon
- Black pepper
- Salt to taste.
- Extra-virgin olive oil
- Rosemary
- Chili
- Rocket salad
- Celery leaves
- 1 shallot
- 1 tablespoon of brown sugar
- 2 tablespoons of red wine
- Extra virgin olive oil
- Salt

Directions:

1. Preparing salmon in a pan is very simple, and just as fast, that's how to proceed: heat a drizzle of extra virgin olive oil in a pan. As soon as the oil is hot, put the salmon steaks in the pan, on the meaty side. Lightly incise the scaly part (the skin), and cook for about 1 minute with sustained heat.

2. Turn them over and cook them also on the skin side. Add the rosemary sprig to the pan and let it take flavor. Salt and pepper slightly and make sure that the skin becomes rusty.

3. Cook for about 2 minutes. While cooking, with the help of a spoon, takes the cooking liquid and pour it on the salmon steaks in order to flavor the whole dish. Once the skin of the salmon steaks has turned golden brown and toasted, remove the pan from the heat. Cut the lemon, lime, and orange into wedges and serve the salmon steaks with freshly prepared citrus wedges, a few sprigs of dill and freshly crushed chili pepper.

4. To prepare the caramelized rocket salad in a pan, start by peeling the shallot and washing the rocket salad thoroughly. Continue taking a non-stick pan, pour a drizzle of olive oil on the bottom, put on the fire, and brown the shallot cut into thin strips for a few minutes.

5. Continue adding the already washed and chopped rocket salad. Sauté the rocket salad for about ten minutes over high heat, then add the brown sugar, wild fennel, and red wine vinegar.

6. Leave to cook for another couple of minutes to reduce the liquid and caramelize the sugar. If necessary, adjust the flavor by adding a pinch of salt and a little more sugar or vinegar. Turn off the heat and let the rocket salad cool in the pan for a few moments before serving.

Nutrition:

- Calories: 120,
- Sodium: 23 mg,
- Dietary Fiber: 2.4 g,
- Total Fat: 2.1 g,
- Total Carbs: 1.3 g,
- Protein: 10.3 g.

38.   Berry Chia Breakfast Bow

Preparation Time: 10 minutes

Cooking time: 0 minute

Servings: 2

Ingredients:

- Eight pitted dates
- 1/2 cup canned coconut milk
- Two tablespoons blanched almonds or raw cashews
- Two teaspoons frozen orange juice concentrate
- One pinch salt
- 1/3 cup almond milk
- 1/2 teaspoon vanilla
- 2 cups diced, strawberries – divided
- 3/4 cup fresh blueberries
- 1/4 cup chia seed
- One small banana, sliced – optional

Directions:

1. In a blender, place dates, coconut milk, almond milk, almonds, orange juice concentrate, cinnamon, salt, and 1 cup strawberries and mix until smooth.
2. Shift mixture to medium bowl and stir in seed chia.
3. Place in the fridge for a minimum of 2 hours, or overnight.
4. Until serving, stir in the blueberries, remaining strawberries (sliced), and sliced bananas. Fresh berries work better than frozen.

Nutrition:

- Calories: 183
- Sodium: 23 mg
- Dietary Fiber: 1.4 g
- Total Fat: 2.1 g
- Total Carbs: 11.3 g

- Protein: 1.3 g

39.   Miso Marinated Baked Cod

Preparation time: 20 minutes

Cooking time: 30 minutes

Serves: 2

Ingredients:

- 1.2 ounces of miso
- 1tablespoon mirin
- 1tablespoon extra virgin olive oil
- 1 Ounce of skinless cod fillet
- 1.3 ounces of red onion, sliced
- 1 clove garlic, finely chopped
- 1.76 ounces of celery, sliced
- 1teaspoon fresh ginger, finely chopped
- One bird's eye chili, finely chopped
- 1.8 ounces of green beans
- Buckwheat
- 1.76 ounces of kale, roughly chopped
- 1teaspoon ground turmeric
- Parsley, roughly chopped
- 1tablespoon tamari or soy sauce
- 1teaspoon sesame seeds

Directions:

1. Heat the oven to 220 ° C/200oC a fan/gas limit of 7.
2. Blend the miso, mirin and 1tsp oil, whisk in the cod and marinate 30 minutes. Transfer to a baking tray, then cook 10 minutes.
3. Meanwhile, heat the remaining oil over a large frying pan. For a few minutes, add the onion and stir-fry, then add the celery, garlic, chili,

ginger, green beans and kale. Keep frying until the kale is tender and cooked through, adding a little water if necessary, to soften the kale.
4. Cook the buckwheat with the turmeric as directed on the box. Attach the parsley, sesame seeds and tamari or soy sauce.
5. Serve to the stir-fry with greens and fish.

Nutrition:

- Calories: 195
- Sodium: 31 mg
- Dietary Fiber: 1.4 g
- Total Fat: 3.1 g
- Total Carbs: 11.3 g
- Protein: 1.3 g

Chapter 5:   Main Meal Recipes

40.   Tuscan Stewed Beans

Preparation time: 20 minutes

Cooking time: 30 minutes

Servings: 1

Ingredients:

- 1 dl. extra virgin olive oil
- Salt to taste
- Pepper as needed.
- Cannellini beans
- Sage
- Garlic clove
- Water

Directions:

1. Soak the beans for at least 12 hours before cooking. Pour the beans in a crockpot with water, a clove of garlic, sage, and a generous pinch of salt, adjust the flame as low as possible.
2. When the water is boiling, cover the pot, and continue cooking for at least 3 and a half hours, taking care that the flame remains very low, the beans in the pot must not move around.
3. Once you are done cooking, serve the beans with extra virgin olive oil, salt, and pepper on the table.

Nutrition:

- Calories: 120,
- Sodium: 23 mg,
- Dietary Fiber: 2.4 g,
- Total Fat: 2.1 g,

- Total Carbs: 1.3 g,
- Protein: 10.3 g.

41.   Buckwheat Tabbouleh With Strawberries

Preparation time: 20 minutes

Cooking time: 30 minutes

Servings: 1

Ingredients:

- Buckwheat (broken)
- Turmeric powder 2 teaspoon
- Avocado 1
- Tomatoes
- Tropea red onions
- Medjool dates (pitted)
- Parsley
- Strawberries
- 2 tablespoons extra virgin olive oil
- Lemon juice 1
- Rocket 1.3 ounce

Direction:

1. Heat up the water to cook the buckwheat.
2. When it boils, add turmeric and buckwheat. Be careful not to overcook it. It is good to leave, it "al dente." When cooked, drain the buckwheat and set aside to cool. Take a large bowl to spice the tabbouleh.
3. Cut the tomatoes into cubes and let them drain for a few minutes in a colander to remove the water.
4. On a cutting board, begin to finely chop the red onion, dates, and parsley and combine them with buckwheat.
5. Peel the avocado and cut it into small cubes and add it with the tomatoes to the buckwheat. Cut the strawberries into slices and gently add them to the rest of the ingredients. Add the chopped arugula, oil, and lemon juice. Mix all the ingredients and let the buckwheat tabbouleh take on extra flavor for an hour before serving it at the table.

Nutrition:

- Calories: 120,
- Sodium: 23 mg,
- Dietary Fiber: 2.4 g,
- Total Fat: 2.1 g,
- Total Carbs: 1.3 g,
- Protein: 10.3 g.

42.   Baked Cod Marinated In Miso With Sautéed Vegetables and Sesame

Preparation time: 20 minutes

Cooking time: 30 minutes

Servings: 1

Ingredients:

- 14 ounces of fish fillets (Mackerel, Cod, etc.)
- 2 spoons of miso
- Vegetables
- Sesame

Directions:

1. Clean the fish fillets, rinse them and dry them well with kitchen paper and mix all the seasonings in a bowl. Spread the sauce on the fish fillets, put them in a plastic bag with zipping (food use) then leave them to marinate in the fridge overnight (*). To cook them, take the fish fillets from the bag, remove the sauce from the fillets using kitchen paper (because this sauce burns easily during cooking)
2. The fish fillet can be roasted in the oven or fried in a pan with a little olive oil.
3. In the case of the oven: grease the grill and arrange the fillets putting the side with the skin down, cook them at 200 ° C for about 8-10 minutes, then turn them and continue to roast for 8-10 minutes
4. In the case of the pan: spread a piece of parchment paper on the pan and arrange the fillets placing the side with the skin down. Cook them on medium heat for 3-4 minutes. After that, turn the fillets and cook over low heat together with the vegetables and sesame with lid for about 10 minutes.

Nutrition:

- Calories 145

- Sodium: 19 mg,
- Dietary Fiber: 5.7 g,
- Total Fat: 12 g,
- Total Carbs: 18 g,
- Protein: 37 g.

43.   Soba in a Miso Broth With Tofu, Celery, and Kale

Preparation time: 20 minutes

Cooking time: 30 minutes

Servings: 1

Ingredients:

- 1l of water
- 4 teaspoons of miso paste
- Noodles 1.3 ounce
- Tofu
- Kale
- Salt
- Pepper

Directions:

1. To prepare the noodles soup, start cutting all the ingredients: then mix and cook the vegetables for about 15 minutes.
2. Add the water flush. Salt and pepper to taste, then to flavor the soup, grate the fresh ginger and cover with a lid to cook the soup over moderate heat for at least 20 minutes, stirring occasionally and adding more water if necessary (you will need to keep the liquid level just above the ingredients).
3. After the necessary time, pour the noodles into the soup and cook for a few minutes (or for the time indicated on the package).
4. At this point, also add the miso paste earlier diluted in a couple of spoonful of warm water, but be careful not to boil the broth because the nutritional properties of the miso are altered.

Nutrition:

- Calories: 220,
- Sodium: 43 mg,
- Dietary Fiber: 5.4 g,
- Total Fat: 2.1 g,

- Total Carbs: 1.3 g,
- Protein: 10.3 g.

44.   Asian King Prawn Stir Fry With Buckwheat Noodles

Preparation Time: 10 minutes

Cooking time: 20 minutes

Servings: 1

Ingredients:

- 2.5 ounces of shelled raw king prawns, deveined
- 2 teaspoons of tamaris
- 1.8 ounces of soba (buckwheat noodles)
- 2 teaspoons extra virgin olive oil
- One garlic clove, finely chopped
- One bird's eye chili, finely chopped
- 1 teaspoon finely chopped fresh ginger
- 1.76 ounces celery, trimmed and sliced
- Red onions, sliced
- Green beans, chopped
- 1.76 ounces of kale, roughly chopped
- Little lovage or celery leaves
- Chicken stock

Directions:

1. Heat a frying pan over a high flame, then cook the prawns for 2–3 minutes in 1 teaspoon tamari and one teaspoon oil. Place the prawns onto a tray. Wipe the pan out with paper from the kitchen, as you will be using it again.
2. Cook the noodles 5–8 minutes in boiling water, or as directed on the packet. Drain and put away.
3. Meanwhile, over medium-high heat, fry the garlic, chili and ginger, red onion, celery, beans and kale in the remaining oil for 2–3 minutes. Add the stock and boil, then cook for one or two minutes until the vegetables are cooked but crunchy.

4. Add the prawns, noodles and leaves of lovage/celery to the pan, bring back to the boil, then remove and eat.

Nutrition:

- Calories: 220,
- Sodium: 43 mg,
- Dietary Fiber: 5.4 g,
- Total Fat: 2.1 g,
- Total Carbs: 1.3 g,
- Protein: 10.3 g.

45.   Fragrant Asian Hotpot

Preparation time: 15 minutes

Cooking time: 45 minutes

Servings: 2

Ingredients:

- 1 teaspoon tomato purée
- 1-star anise, crushed (or 1/4 teaspoon ground anise)
- Small handful parsley, stalks finely chopped
- Juice of 1/2 lime
- Small handful coriander, stalks finely chopped
- 500ml chicken stock, fresh or made with one cube
- 1/2 carrot, peeled and cut
- Beansprouts
- Broccoli, cut into small florets
- 1 tablespoon good-quality miso paste
- 3.5 ounces of raw tiger prawns
- 1.76 ounces of rice noodles that are cooked according to packet instructions
- Cooked water chestnuts, drained
- 3.5 ounces of firm tofu, chopped
- Little Sushi ginger, chopped

Directions:

1. In a large saucepan, put the tomato purée, star anise, parsley stalks, coriander stalks, lime juice, and chicken stock and bring to boil for 10 minutes.
2. Stir in the carrot, broccoli, prawns, tofu, noodles and water chestnuts and cook gently until the prawns are cooked. Take it from heat and stir in the ginger sushi and the paste miso.
3. Serve sprinkled with peregrine leaves and coriander.

Nutrition:

- Calories: 220,
- Sodium: 43 mg,
- Dietary Fiber: 5.4 g,
- Total Fat: 2.1 g,
- Total Carbs: 1.3 g,
- Protein: 10.3 g.

46.   Red Onion Dhal

Preparation time: 10 minutes

Cooking time: 10 minutes

Servings: 1

Ingredient:

- 1 teaspoon extra virgin olive oil
- 1 teaspoon mustard seeds
- 1.5oz red onion, finely chopped
- 1 garlic clove, finely chopped
- 1 teaspoon finely chopped fresh ginger
- 1 bird's eye chili, finely chopped
- 1 teaspoon mild curry powder
- 2 teaspoon ground turmeric
- 300ml vegetable stock
- 1.4oz red lentils, rinsed
- 2.3oz kale
- 50ml tinned coconut milk
- 1.4oz buckwheat

Directions:

1. In a moderately sized saucepan, warm the olive oil over a medium heat. Toss in the mustard seeds and fry until they start to crackle. Add the garlic, ginger, chili, and onion frying for 10 minutes, or until the onion is tender.
2. Throw in 1 tsp turmeric and curry powder, and then stir. Cook for a few minutes until fragrant, then pour in the stock and bring to the boil. Pour in the lentils and cook for 30 minutes.
3. Add the coconut milk and kale, cooking for another 5 minutes or so. As the dhal is brewing, rinse the buckwheat with water and cook it according to packet instructions. Drain and serve with the dhal.

Nutrition:

- Calories: 295
- Sodium: 30 mg
- Dietary Fiber: 1.4 g
- Total Fat: 4.3 g
- Total Carbs: 16.3 g
- Protein: 1.4 g

47.   Coq Au Vin

Preparation Time: 10 minutes

Cooking Time: 15 minutes

Servings: 8

Ingredients:

- 1 lb button mushrooms
- 2 ounces of streaky bacon, chopped
- 16 chicken thighs, skin removed
- 3 cloves of garlic, crushed
- 3 tablespoons fresh parsley, chopped
- 3 carrots, chopped
- 2 red onions, chopped
- 2 tablespoons plain flour
- 2 tablespoons olive oil
- 1¼ pints red wine
- 1 bouquet grain

Directions:

1. On a large plate, put the flour and coat the chicken in it. Heat the olive oil, then add the chicken and brown it, before setting aside.
2. Fry the bacon in the pan, then add the onion and cook for 5 minutes.
3. Pour in the red wine and add the chicken, carrots, bouquet grain, and garlic. Transfer it to a large ovenproof dish.
4. Cook at 180C/360F for an hour.
5. Remove the bouquet grain and skim off any excess fat, if necessary.
6. Add in the mushrooms and cook for 15 minutes.
7. Stir in the parsley just before serving.

Nutrition:

- Calories: 220,
- Sodium: 43 mg,

- Dietary Fiber: 5.4 g,
- Total Fat: 2.1 g,
- Total Carbs: 1.3 g,
- Protein: 10.3 g.

48.   Turkey Satay Skewers

Preparation Time: 10 minutes

Cooking Time: 15 minutes

Servings: 2

Ingredients:

- 9 ounces of turkey breast, cubed
- 1 ounce of smooth peanut butter
- 1 clove of garlic, crushed
- ½ small bird's eye chili or more if you like it hotter, finely chopped
- ½ teaspoon ground turmeric
- 7fl oz. coconut milk
- 2 teaspoons soy sauce

Directions:

1. Combine the coconut milk, peanut butter, turmeric, soy sauce, garlic and chili.
2. Add the turkey pieces to the bowl and stir them until they are completely coated.
3. Push the turkey onto metal skewers.
4. Place the satay skewers on a barbeque or under a hot grill broiler and cook for 4-5 minutes on each side, until they are completely cooked.

Nutrition:

- Calories: 220,
- Sodium: 43 mg,
- Dietary Fiber: 5.4 g,
- Total Fat: 2.1 g,
- Total Carbs: 1.3 g,
- Protein: 10.3 g.

49.   Salmon & Capers

Preparation Time: 10 minutes

Cooking Time: 15 minutes

Servings: 4

Ingredients:

- 3 ounces of Greek yogurt
- 4 salmon fillets, skin removed
- 4 teaspoons Dijon Mustard
- 1 tablespoon capers, chopped
- 2 teaspoons fresh parsley
- Zest of 1 lemon

Directions:

1. Put the yogurt, mustard, lemon zest, parsley, and capers in a mixing bowl. Thoroughly coat the salmon in the mixture.
2. Place the salmon under a hot grill broiler and cook for 3-4 minutes on each side, or until the fish is cooked.
3. Serve with mashed potatoes and vegetables or a large green leafy salad.

Nutrition:

- Calories: 220,
- Sodium: 43 mg,
- Dietary Fiber: 5.4 g,
- Total Fat: 2.1 g,
- Total Carbs: 1.3 g,
- Protein: 10.3 g.

50.   Chili Con Carne

Preparation Time: 10 minutes

Cooking Time: 15 minutes

Servings: 4

Ingredients:

- 15 ounces of lean minced beef
- 14 ounces of chopped tomatoes
- 7 ounces of red kidney beans
- 2 tablespoons tomato purée
- 2 cloves of garlic, crushed
- 2 red onions, chopped
- 2 bird's-eye chilies, finely chopped
- 1 red pepper bell pepper, chopped
- 1 stick of celery, finely chopped
- 1 tablespoon cumin
- 1 tablespoon turmeric
- 1 tablespoon cocoa powder
- 14 FL oz. beef stock broth
- 6fl oz. red wine
- 1 tablespoon olive oil

Directions:

1. Put the oil in a saucepan, then add the onion and cook for 5 minutes.
2. Add in the garlic, celery, chili, turmeric, and cumin and cook for 2 minutes before adding then meat then cook for another 5 minutes.
3. Pour in the stock broth, red wine, tomatoes, tomato purée, red pepper, bell pepper, kidney beans, and cocoa powder.
4. Let it simmer for 45 minutes, keep it covered, and stirring occasionally.
5. Serve with brown rice or buckwheat.

Nutrition:

- Calories: 220,
- Sodium: 43 mg,
- Dietary Fiber: 5.4 g,
- Total Fat: 2.1 g,
- Total Carbs: 1.3 g,
- Protein: 10.3 g.

51.   Prawn & Coconut Curry

Preparation Time: 10 minutes

Cooking Time: 15 minutes

Servings: 4

Ingredients:

- 14 ounces of tinned chopped tomatoes
- 14 ounces of large prawns' shrimps, shelled and raw
- 1 ounce of fresh coriander cilantro, chopped
- 3 red onions, finely chopped
- 3 cloves of garlic, crushed
- 2 bird's eye chilies
- ½ teaspoon ground coriander cilantro
- ½ teaspoon turmeric
- 14fl oz. coconut milk
- 1 tablespoon olive oil
- Juice of 1 lime

Directions:

1. Place the onions, garlic, tomatoes, chilies, lime juice, turmeric, ground coriander, chilies and half of the fresh coriander cilantro into a blender and blitz until you have a smooth curry paste.
2. In a frying pan, put the oil, add the paste and cook for 2 minutes.
3. Stir in the coconut milk and warm it thoroughly.
4. Add the prawn's shrimps to the paste and cook them until they have turned pink and are completely cooked.
5. Stir in the fresh coriander cilantro. Serve with rice.

Nutrition:

- Calories: 220,
- Sodium: 43 mg,
- Dietary Fiber: 5.4 g,
- Total Fat: 2.1 g,

- Total Carbs: 1.3 g,
- Protein: 10.3 g.

52.   Fried Cauliflower Rice

Preparation time: 20 minutes

Cooking time: 40 minutes

Servings: 1

Ingredients:

- A piece of cauliflower
- A spoonful of coconut oil
- Cut red onion
- Garlic clove
- Vegetable soup
- Fresh ginger
- Teaspoon paprika
- 1/2 carrot slices
- 1/2 sliced red pepper
- 1/2 slice of lemon juice
- Pumpkin seed spoon

Directions:

1. New coriander preparation spoon:
2. Cut the cauliflower into millet seeds in a food processor.
3. Cut onions, garlic and ginger, sliced carrots, peppers, and chopped herbs.
4. Add 1 tablespoon of coconut oil to the pan to melt it, then add half the onion and garlic to the pan and fry briefly until transparent.
5. Add cauliflower rice and season with salt.
6. Pour the broth and stir until evaporated. Then the cauliflower rice becomes soft.
7. Remove the rice from the pan and set it aside.
8. Dissolve the remaining coconut oil in the pan, then add onion, garlic, ginger, carrot, and remaining pepper.

9. Saute for a few minutes until the vegetables are tender. Season with a little salt.

10.   Add the cauliflower rice again, heat the whole plate, and add the lemon juice.

11.   Decorate with pumpkin seeds and coriander before serving.

Nutrition:

- Calories: 210,
- Sodium: 23 mg,
- Dietary Fiber: 6.4 g,
- Total Fat: 2.1 g,
- Total Carbs: 2.3 g,
- Protein: 10.3 g.

53.   Miso-Marinated Baked Cod With Stir-Fried Greens and Sesame

Preparation time: 20 minutes

Cooking time: 40 minutes

Servings: 1

Ingredients:

- One tablespoon of extra virgin olive oil
- 3 1/2 teaspoons of miso
- One tablespoon of mirin
- 1/8 cup of a red onion, sliced
- 1 x 7-ounce of skinless cod fillet
- Two garlic cloves, finely chopped
- 3/8 cup of celery, sliced
- One teaspoon of finely chopped fresh ginger
- One Thai chili, finely chopped
- 3/4 cup of kale, roughly chopped
- 3/8 cup of green beans
- Two tablespoons of parsley, roughly chopped
- One teaspoon of sesame seeds
- 1/4 cup of buckwheat
- One tablespoon of tamari (or soy sauce, if not avoiding gluten)
- One teaspoon of ground turmeric

Directions:

1. Combine the miso, mirin, and one teaspoon of olive oil. Rub the mix all over the whole cod and set for 30 minutes to marinate. Oven heated to 220 degrees C (425 degrees F).
2. Bake the cod for 10 minutes.
3. Heat up the remaining oil in a large frying pan or wok. Add the celery, garlic, chili, ginger, green beans, and kale and fry for a few minutes. Turn

until the kale is soft and cooked. To help the cooking process, you might have to put a bit of water into the pot.

4. Cook buckwheat together with turmeric following the package instructions.

5. Serve the stir-fry with sesame, parsley, tamari seeds, and fish. Serve in the stir-fry.

Nutrition:

- Calories: 210,
- Sodium: 23 mg,
- Dietary Fiber: 6.4 g,
- Total Fat: 2.1 g,
- Total Carbs: 2.3 g,
- Protein: 10.3 g.

54.   Calamarata With Squid, Capers and Lemon

Preparation time: 10 Minutes,

Cooking time: 2 Minutes,

Servings: 4

Ingredients:

- 2 clean squid
- 1 handful of salted capers
- 1 shallot
- 1 untreated lemon
- A few sprigs of thyme
- 1/2 glass of white wine
- Calamari

Directions:

1. Clean the squid, removing skin, eyes and mouth, then cut them into very thin rings.
2. Cut the shallot into slices and brown it in a pan with a little oil.
3. Then add the squid and cook over high heat, then blend with the wine and dry.
4. Add the rinsed capers well and cook with a spoonful of water.
5. While cooking the Calamarata, cut the lemon peel into julienne strips, taking care to remove the white part.
6. Drain the pasta and sauté over high heat for a few moments, then add the lemon and raw oil. Serve hot, perfuming with fresh thyme.

Nutrition:

- Calories: 123
- Sodium: 27 mg
- Dietary Fiber: 1.4 g
- Total Fat: 2.1 g
- Total Carbs: 12.3 g
- Protein: 1.6 g

55.   Asian Shrimp Stir-Fry With Buckwheat Noodles

Preparation time: 20 minutes

Cooking time: 40 minutes

Servings: 1

Ingredients:

- 2 teaspoons of tamari (you can use soy sauce if you are not avoiding gluten)
- 1/3 pound of shelled raw jumbo shrimp, deveined
- 2 teaspoons of extra virgin olive oil
- 2 garlic cloves, finely chopped
- 3 ounces of soba (buckwheat noodles)
- One teaspoon of finely chopped fresh ginger
- One Thai chili, finely chopped
- 1/2 cup of celery, including leaves, trimmed and sliced, with leaves set aside
- 1/8 cup of red onions, sliced
- 3/4 cup of kale, roughly chopped
- 1/2 cup of green beans, chopped
- 1/2 cup of chicken stock

Directions:

1. Prepare the pan on high heat, then cook the shrimps for 2 to 3 minutes with 1 tamari teaspoon and one olive oil teaspoon.
2. Switch to a tray of shrimp. Cover the pan with a towel or cloth, and you'll need it again.
3. Cook the noodles for 5 to 8 minutes or as indicated on the box in boiling water. Drain and reserve.
4. Fry the garlic, pepper, the ginger, and red onion, celery (but not the blade) over half to high heat for 2 to 3 minutes in the remaining tamari

and oil. Stir in the stock and boil until they are tender but crunchy, then simmer for a minute or two.

5. Stir in a pan and put back to boil, then take the shrimp, pasta, and celery leaves from the oven, and eat.

Nutrition:

- Calories: 210,
- Sodium: 23 mg,
- Dietary Fiber: 6.4 g,
- Total Fat: 2.1 g,
- Total Carbs: 2.3 g,
- Protein: 10.3 g.

56.   Strawberry Buckwheat Tabbouleh

Preparation time: 20 minutes

Cooking time: 40 minutes

Servings: 1

Ingredients:

- 1 tablespoon of ground turmeric
- 1/3 cup of buckwheat
- 1/2 cup of avocado
- 1/8 cup of red onion
- 3/8 cup of tomato
- 1 tablespoon of capers
- 1/8 cup of Medjool dates, pitted
- 2/3 cup of strawberries, hulled
- 3/4 cup of parsley
- Juice of 1/2 a lemon
- 1 tablespoon of extra virgin olive oil
- 1 ounce of arugula

Directions:

1. Cook the buckwheat with the turmeric according to the directions on the box.
2. Rinse and drain to cool off.
3. Chop the tomato finely, peppers, red onions, dates, capers, and pots, and mix along with the fresh buckwheat.
4. Dice the strawberries and combine the oils with the lemon juice softly in the salad. Serve on arugula bed.

Nutrition:

- Calories: 210,
- Sodium: 23 mg,
- Dietary Fiber: 6.4 g,
- Total Fat: 2.1 g,

- Total Carbs: 2.3 g,
- Protein: 10.3 g.

57.   Date and Walnut Cinnamon Bites

Preparation time: 5 Minutes

Cooking time: 0 minutes

Serving: 1

Ingredients:

- Three pitted Medjool dates
- Three walnut halves
- Add the ground cinnamon, to taste

Directions:

1. Split each walnut half carefully into three pieces and then do the same with the dates.
2. Place on top of every date a piece of walnut and cover with cinnamon dust.

Nutrition:

- Calories: 210,
- Sodium: 23 mg,
- Dietary Fiber: 6.4 g,
- Total Fat: 2.1 g,
- Total Carbs: 2.3 g,
- Protein: 10.3 g.

58. Oriental Salmon and Broccoli Traybake

Preparation time: 10 Minutes,

Cooking time: 30 Minutes,

Servings: 4

Ingredients:

- One head of broccoli, broken into florets
- 4 skins-on salmon fillets
- Juice ½ lemon, ½ lemon quartered
- 2 tablespoons of soy sauce
- Small bunch spring onions, sliced

Directions:

1. 180C/160C heating stove/gas
2. Place the salmon in a large tin to roast, making space for each fillet.
3. Wash and dry broccoli and arrange around the fillets, while still a little wet. Sprinkle the lemon juice on top, then apply the quarter of a lemon.
4. Sprinkle half the onions with a little olive oil on top and add them to the oven for 14 minutes.
5. Remove from the oven, sprinkle it with the soy, and return to the oven for another 4 minutes before the salmon is ready. Just before serving, sprinkle with the remaining spring onions.

Nutrition:

- Calories: 210,
- Sodium: 23 mg,
- Dietary Fiber: 6.4 g,
- Total Fat: 2.1 g,
- Total Carbs: 2.3 g,
- Protein: 10.3 g.

59.   Fusilli Pasta With Cherry Tomatoes, Capers and Crunchy Crumbs

Preparation time: 10 Minutes,

Cooking time: 40 Minutes,

Servings: 4

Ingredients:

- Whole meal bread
- Salted capers
- 1 clove of garlic
- 1 hot pepper
- Oblong cherry tomatoes
- Extra virgin olive oil
- Salt
- Fusilli

Directions:

1. To make the fusilli with cherry tomatoes, capers and crunchy crumbs, start putting a pot of slightly salted water on the fire to boil the pasta. So, dedicate yourself to seasoning.
2. Chop the bread and put it in a hot pan together with the desalted capers, the clove of garlic and the chili pepper. Toast stirring often so that it is uniformly colored without burning.
3. Cut the cherry tomatoes in half and remove the seeds. Arrange them in a colander, add a pinch of salt and let them lose the excess vegetable water.
4. Remove the garlic clove and transfer the toast with the capers and the chili pepper into the mixer. Cut into crumbs.
5. Put everything back in a pan on high heat and give it one last toast to take a nice brown color, obviously without burning.
6. Heat 3 or 4 tablespoons of oil in a pan and add the cherry tomatoes that you will sauté for a few seconds over a high flame.

7. Drain the al dente fusilli, add them to the cherry tomatoes and sauté for a minute.
8. Divide into individual dishes, finish with a generous sprinkling of bread, and a round of oil as desired. Serve your fusilli with cherry tomatoes, capers and crunchy crumbs immediately.

Nutrition:

- Calories: 210,
- Sodium: 23 mg,
- Dietary Fiber: 6.4 g,
- Total Fat: 2.1 g,
- Total Carbs: 2.3 g,
- Protein: 10.3 g.

60.   Pan-Fried Aubergine Olives and Capers

Preparation time: 10 Minutes,

Cooking time: 20 Minutes,

Servings: 4

Ingredients:

- 5 tomatoes
- 2 onions
- 2 cloves of garlic
- 1 tablespoon of pitted Taggiasca olives
- 1 tablespoon of salted capers
- A sprig of parsley
- Extra virgin olive oil
- 1 tablespoon of vinegar
- 1 teaspoon of sugar
- Salt
- Black pepper
- 4 small Aubergine

Directions:

1. To make the Aubergine in a pan with olives and capers, start washing and drying the Aubergine.
2. Cut them into cubes after removing the central part, which is particularly rich in seeds. Leave them in salt for half an hour to lose some of their bitter water.
3. After half an hour, rinse the Aubergine cubes and dry them. In a saucepan, heat two Cachia of oil, add the onions, cut in icing and the whole cloves of garlic.
4. When they are slightly golden, remove the cloves of garlic and add the Aubergine cubes, then add the fresh tomatoes, seeded and diced: salt and pepper.

5. Cook over medium heat for about a quarter of an hour, stirring frequently so that eggplants and tomatoes do not stick to the bottom of the pan.
6. Now add the finely chopped parsley, olives, capers rinsed of salt and squeezed, vinegar and sugar.
7. Let it flavor well and then taste the Aubergine to check that they have a sweet and sour taste: if they were too sour, add a pinch of sugar, if they were too sweet add a splash of vinegar.
8. After a few minutes, remove from the heat: you can serve the eggplants in a pan with olives and warm or lukewarm capers.

Nutrition:

- Calories: 270
- Sodium: 13 mg
- Dietary Fiber: 6.4 g
- Total Fat: 3.1 g
- Total Carbs: 213
- Protein: 10.3 g

61.   Salmon With Caper Butter

Preparation time: 10 Minutes,

Cooking time: 20 Minutes,

Servings: 4

Ingredients:

- 2 tablespoons of salted capers
- Extra virgin olive oil,salt, black pepper
- 4 salmon steaks
- Butter

Directions:

1. To prepare the salmon with caper butter, first rinse and dry the salmon steaks, then place them in a pan where you have heated two tablespoons of oil.
2. Cook them on both sides, over medium heat, for 6-7 minutes and towards the end of the cooking season with salt and pepper.
3. In the meantime, let the butter melt in a saucepan over low heat and without frying it. Season the desalted and well-dried capers for a couple of minutes.
4. When the salmon steaks are cooked, transfer them to the serving dish.
5. Sprinkle the fish with the flavored melted butter and serve immediately your salmon steaks with caper butter.

Nutrition:

- Calories: 270
- Sodium: 13 mg
- Dietary Fiber: 6.4 g
- Total Fat: 3.1 g
- Total Carbs: 213 g
- Protein: 10.3 g

62.   Chicken and Kale Curry

Preparation time: 10 minutes

Cooking time: 20 minutes

Servings: 1

Ingredients:

- 1.5 cups boneless, skinless chicken thigh, raw and cut into bite-sized pieces
- ½ tablespoon olive oil
- 1 tablespoon turmeric powder
- 1 whole, diced red onion
- 2 cloves of garlic, crushed and minced
- 1 bird's eye chili, minced remove seeds if you prefer something less spicy
- ½ tablespoon fresh ginger root, chopped
- ½ tablespoon curry powder (more to taste if you prefer it spicier)
- 1 cardamom pods
- 1/3 cup light coconut milk from a can (make sure it is the cooking kind, not the drinking milk substitute kind)
- ½ of a 14oz can have chopped tomato
- ½ of a 14oz can of chicken stock
- Cilantro for garnish

Directions:

1. In a glass bowl, add your chicken, 1 teaspoon of oil, and 1 tsp of turmeric. Combine, mix, and let it marinate. Use a spoon if you do not want stained fingers. Leave it in the fridge for at least 30 minutes.
2. Cook the chicken over medium heat in a frying pan for 5 minutes until it is browned. Place chicken in a clean bowl and set aside. Do not put the chicken back into the bowl, it was in when it was raw.
3. Heat 1 teaspoon of olive oil at medium heat and add in the onion, garlic, chili, and ginger.
4. Cook it for ten minutes and turn on some ventilation—this will get spicy!

133

5. Add in the curry powder and 2 tsp of turmeric—Cook for another minute.
6. Mix in the canned tomatoes, coconut milk, cardamom pods, and ½ can of chicken stock. Reduce heat to barely above a simmer and wait 30 minutes
7. When the sauce is reduced, add the chicken and kale. Cook until kale has begun to wilt.
8. Serve over rice or buckwheat. Top it with a sprinkling of chopped cilantro.

Nutrition:

- Calories: 210
- Sodium: 13 mg
- Dietary Fiber: 6.4 g
- Total Fat: 3.1 g
- Total Carbs: 213 g
- Protein: 2.3 g

63.   Old Chicken Roll

Preparation time: 10 minutes

Cooking time: 10 minutes

Servings: 2

Ingredients:

- Egg
- Almond milk
- 1 teaspoon olive oil (delicate)
- 1 teaspoon of Celtic sea salt
- Tapioca flour
- Prepare 3 tablespoons of coconut flour, 10 chicken breasts, and mixed salad 2 hands

Directions:

1. Beat the eggs in a bowl, then add almond milk, olive oil and salt.
2. Add cassava flour and coconut flour and mix until the dough is even.
3. Grease the pan, then pour 1/6 of the dough into the pan.
4. The diameter of the package should be about 15 cm.
5. Fry the skin on both sides until golden.
6. Repeat this step for the rest of the dough.
7. You can wrap the chicken in it, or add other salads or raw vegetables as needed.

Nutrition:

- Calories: 104
- Sodium: 33 mg
- Dietary Fiber: 1.4 g
- Total Fat: 4.1 g
- Total Carbs: 16.3 g
- Protein: 1.3 g

64.   Chicken and Bean Casserole

Preparation time: 15 minutes

Cooking time: 55 minutes

Servings: 4

Ingredients:

- 400g chopped tomatoes
- 400g tinned cannellini beans or haricot beans
- 8 chicken thighs, skin removed
- 2 carrots, peeled and finely chopped
- 2 red onions, chopped
- 4 sticks of celery
- 4 large mushrooms
- 2 red peppers (bell peppers), de-seeded and chopped
- 1 clove of garlic
- 2 teaspoons soy sauce
- 1 olive oil
- 1.75 liters chicken stock (broth)

Directions:

1. Heat the olive oil in a saucepan, add the garlic and onions and cook for 5 minutes.
2. Add in the chicken and cook for 5 minutes then add the carrots, cannellini beans, celery, red peppers (bell peppers) and mushrooms.
3. Pour in the stock (broth) soy sauce and tomatoes.
4. Bring it to the boil, reduce the heat and simmer for 45 minutes.
5. Serve with rice or new potatoes.

Nutrition:

- Calories: 509
- Net carbs: 12.5g
- Fat: 6.5g

- Fiber: 1.1g
- Protein: 27.4g

65.   Apple and Cinnamon Rolls

Preparation time: 10 minutes

Cooking time: 10 minutes

Servings: 2

Ingredients:

- 2 Eggs (stir)
- 240 ml of almond milk
- Teaspoon olive oil (delicate)
- 1 teaspoon Celtic sea salt
- Tapioca flour
- 1 spoon of coconut flour is used for decoration
- 1 tablespoon clarified butter
- 1 teaspoon cinnamon
- 1 cranberry in hand
- Prepare a teaspoon of lemon juice

Directions:

1. Beat the eggs in a bowl, then add almond milk, olive oil and salt.
2. Add cassava flour and coconut flour and mix until the dough is even.
3. Grease the pan, then pour 1/6 of the dough into the pan.
4. The diameter of the package should be about 15 cm.
5. Fry the skin on both sides until golden.
6. Heat the clarified butter in the pan.
7. Add diced apples, cinnamon, blueberries and lemon juice and cook over medium heat until the apples are soft.
8. Place a spoonful of apples on the wrapping paper and fold it into rolls.
9. Please enjoy!

Nutrition:

- Calories: 104,
- Sodium: 33 mg,

- Dietary Fiber: 1.4 g,
- Total Fat: 4.1 g,
- Total Carbs: 16.3 g,
- Protein: 1.3 g.

66.   Spinach and Eggplant Casserole

Preparation time: 20 minutes

Cooking time: 30 minutes

Servings: 1

Ingredients:

- Eggplant
- Onion slices
- 1 spoon of olive oil
- 450 g spinach (fresh)
- 1 Tomato
- Egg
- Almond milk
- 1 teaspoon lemon juice
- Almond flour preparation spoon

Directions:

1. Preheat the oven to 200 ° C.
2. Thinly slice eggplant, onion and tomato, and sprinkle some salt on the eggplant.
3. Brush the eggplant and onions with olive oil and fry them in the pan.
4. Place spinach in a large pot, heat over medium heat, then drain the colander.
5. Put the vegetables in a frying pan: first eggplant, then spinach, then onions and tomatoes. Repeat again
6. Beat eggs with almond milk, lemon juice, salt and pepper, then pour them on the vegetables.
7. Sprinkle almond flour on a plate and bake for about 30 to 40 minutes.

Nutrition:

- Calories: 104
- Sodium: 23 mg

- Dietary Fiber: 1.3 g
- Total Fat: 4.2 g
- Total Carbs: 15.3 g
- Protein: 1.4 g

67. Butterfly Ebi

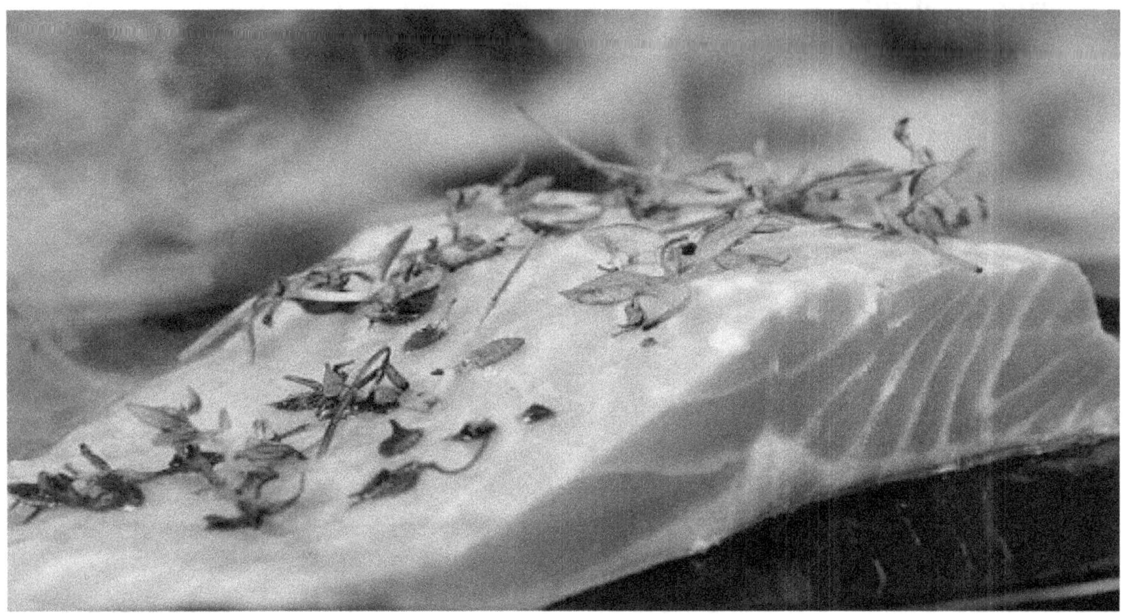

Preparation time: 10 Minutes

Cooking time: 40 Minutes

Servings: 4

Ingredients:

- 20 medium-sized fresh purple prawns
- 1 yellow carrot
- 1 purple carrot
- 1 orange carrot
- Capers
- 10 green daikon sprouts
- Extra virgin olive oil for cooking
- Fine salt
- For marinating:
- Rice vinegar

- Mirin (sweet cooking sake)
- Dashi (fish broth)
- Sugar
- Salt
- For the extraction:
- Yellow carrot extraction
- Ginger extraction
- Sansho (a variety of Japanese pepper)
- Agar
- For the application:
- Sake
- Mirin
- For the chips:
- Prawn pulp

Directions:

1. Clean the prawns keeping only the tail, peel and cut the carrots to a thickness of 1mm.
2. Bring all the marinating ingredients to a boil and then dip the carrots color by color, keeping them separate and marinate them for 1 minute. Drain and roll them one by one, being careful to keep the shape.
3. Spend extractor cutouts of yellow carrots. Bring the juice obtained to a boil to remove all impurities, add the other ingredients and boil for 20 seconds. Let it cool down. Once cold and solid, blend everything, making it a homogeneous and shiny cream. Desalinate the capers under water for 20 minutes. Boil them in sake and mirin until complete reduction of the liquid. Spread the shrimp meat on the silpat and season with the sansho. Dry it in the oven at 70 degrees for at least 18 hours. In a very hot pan, sauté the purple prawns with the extra virgin olive oil and a pinch of salt for 20 seconds. Compose the dish.

Nutrition:

- Calories: 270

- Sodium: 13 mg
- Dietary Fiber: 6.4 g
- Total Fat: 3.1 g
- Total Carbs: 213 g
- Protein: 10.3 g

68.   Tofu And Curry

Preparation time: 10 minutes

Cooking time: 30 minutes

Servings: 1

Ingredients:

- 8 ounces dried lentils (preferably red)
- 1 cup of boiling water
- 1 cup frozen Edamame beans
- 7 oz. (1/2 of most packages) firm tofu, diced
- 2 tomatoes, chopped
- 1 lime juice
- 5-6 kale leaves, stems removed and torn
- 1 large onion, chopped
- 4 garlic cloves, peeled and grated
- 1 large piece of grated ginger
- 1/2 red pepper, seeded (use less if too much)
- 1/2 teaspoon ground turmeric
- 1/4 teaspoon cayenne pepper
- 1 teaspoon paprika
- 1/2 teaspoon ground cumin
- 1 teaspoon of salt
- 1 tablespoon olive oil

Directions:

1. Add the onion, sauté in the oil for a few minutes, then add the chili, garlic and ginger a little longer until they wilt, but do not burn. Add the spices, lentils and stir.
2. Add boiling water and boil for 10 minutes. Simmer for up to 30 minutes so that it is braised but not too mushy. However, you need to check the texture of the lenses in half.

3. Add the tomatoes, tofu and edamame, then the lime juice and the kale. Try when the kale is tender and ready to serve.

Nutrition:

- Calories: 495
- Sodium: 31 mg
- Dietary Fiber: 1.6 g
- Total Fat: 4.2 g
- Total Carbs: 14.3 g
- Protein: 1.4 g

69.   Miso Sesame Chicken

Preparation time: 10 minutes

Cooking time: 10 minutes

Servings: 1

Ingredients:

- 1 skinless cod fillet
- ½ cup buckwheat
- ½ red onion, sliced
- 2 Celery stalks, sliced
- 10 green beans
- 2 Cups of chopped kale
- 3 Parsley sprigs
- 1 clove of garlic, finely chopped
- 1 pinch of cayenne pepper or ½ chili pepper
- 1 teaspoon fresh ginger, finely chopped
- 1 A teaspoon of sesame seeds
- 2 Teaspoon of miso
- 1 tablespoon. Mirin/rice wine vinegar
- 1 tablespoon. Extra virgin olive oil
- 1 tablespoon. Soy sauce 1 teaspoon ground turmeric

Direction:

1. Cover the cod with a mixture of miso, mirin and 1 teaspoon of oil and keep in the refrigerator for 30 minutes to an hour.
2. Heat the oven to 400 F and cook the cod for 10 minutes.
3. Sauté the onion and sauté in the remaining oil with the green beans, kale, celery, chili, garlic and ginger. Sauté until kale is wilted, but beans and celery are tender. Add drops of water to the pan if necessary.
4. Cook the turmeric buckwheat for 3 minutes, depending on the package. Put the sesame, parsley and tamari in the sauce and serve with vegetables and fish.

Nutrition:

- Calories: 125
- Sodium: 32 mg
- Dietary Fiber: 1.3 g
- Total Fat: 4.3 g
- Total Carbs: 16.2 g
- Protein: 1.2 g

70.   Chicken and Kale With Hot Sauce

Preparation time: 10 minutes

Cooking time: 30 minutes

Servings: 1

Ingredients:

- 1 boneless, skinless chicken breast/breast
- ¼ cup buckwheat
- Lemon in the juice
- 1 tablespoon. Extra virgin olive oil
- 1 cup chopped kale
- 1/2 red onion, sliced
- 1 Teaspoon fresh ginger, chopped
- 2 Teaspoon ground turmeric
- Sauce
- 1 tomato
- 3 sprigs of chopped parsley
- 1 tablespoon chopped capers
- 1 chili pepper, seeded and chopped (use less if desired)
- Lemon juice

Direction:

1. Chop all of the above ingredients just for the sauce and store-in a bowl.
2. Heat the oven at 425 F.
3. Add a teaspoon of turmeric, lemon juice and a little chicken oil, cover and set aside for 10 minutes.
4. Put the chicken and marinade in a hot pan and cook for 2 to 3 minutes on each side to burn them. Then slide everything onto a baking sheet and bake for about 20 minutes or until it is cooked (pink proof).
5. Lightly steam kale in a steamer or on the stove with a lid and a little water for about 5 minutes. You want to wither, not cook or burn kale.

6. Sauté the red onions and ginger and after 4-5 minutes, add the cooked kale and stir for 1 minute.
7. Boil the buckwheat and add the turmeric (see pack or look online if you bought in bulk for how to cook). Serve the chicken with buckwheat, kale and hot sauce.

Nutrition:

- Calories: 295
- Sodium: 31 mg
- Dietary Fiber: 1.2 g
- Total Fat: 2.1 g
- Total Carbs: 14.3 g
- Protein: 1.6 g

71.   Sirtfood Cauliflower Couscous & Turkey Steak

Preparation time: 10 minutes

Cooking time: 30 minutes

Servings: 1

Ingredients:

- 2oz cauliflower, roughly chopped
- 1 garlic clove, finely chopped
- 1.3oz red onion, finely chopped
- 1 bird's eye chili, finely chopped
- 1 teaspoon finely chopped fresh ginger
- 2 tablespoons extra-virgin olive oil
- 2 teaspoons ground turmeric
- 1.2oz sun-dried tomatoes, finely chopped
- 0.7oz parsley
- 2.3oz turkey steak
- 1 teaspoon dried sage
- Juice of ½ lemon
- 1 tablespoon capers

Direction:

1. Disintegrate the cauliflower using a food processor. Blend in 1-2 pulses until the cauliflower has a breadcrumb-like consistency.
2. In a skillet, fry garlic, chili, ginger and red onion in 1 tsp olive oil for 2-3 minutes. Throw in the turmeric and cauliflower, then cook for another 1-2 minutes. Remove from heat and add the tomatoes and roughly half the parsley.
3. Garnish the turkey steak with sage and dress with oil. In a skillet, over medium heat, fry the turkey steak for 5 minutes, turning occasionally. Once the steak is cooked, add lemon juice, capers and a dash of water. Stir and serve with the couscous.

Nutrition:

- Calories: 195
- Sodium: 31 mg
- Dietary Fiber: 1.4 g
- Total Fat: 4.3 g
- Total Carbs: 16.4 g
- Protein: 1.3 g

72.   Mushroom Scramble

Preparation time: 10 minutes

Cooking time: 10 minutes

Servings: 1

Ingredients:

- 4 eggs
- 2 teaspoons turmeric (ground)
- 3 teaspoons curry powder
- 2/3 cups chopped kale
- 2 teaspoons olive oil (extra virgin)
- 1 bird's eye chili, sliced (remove seeds if you prefer less burn)
- Button mushrooms, sliced up just a handful or two
- 1/3 cup of parsley, chopped.

Directions:

1. Combine the turmeric and curry powder in a small bowl. Add a small amount of water and mix until it creates a paste
2. In a pot, steam your kale for just a few minutes—no more than 3
3. Heat the oil up on medium in a frying pan. Then, sauté the mushroom slices and the pepper slices. Wait for the mushrooms to start to soften.
4. Then, crack the eggs into the pan and mix with the spice paste. Cook the whole thing over medium heat for a minute and then mix in the kale.
5. Cook for another minute or until eggs are fully cooked. Then add the parsley to the pan, mix together to combine, and serve.

Nutrition:

- Calories: 216
- Sodium: 26 mg
- Dietary Fiber: 1.2 g
- Total Fat: 4.6 g
- Total Carbs: 16.2 g
- Protein: 1.4 g

73.   Vegetarian Curry

Preparation time: 20 minutes

Cooking time: 30 minutes

Servings: 1

Ingredients:

- Radish
- Onion slices
- Clove garlic
- Spoon curry powder
- Teaspoon coriander (ground)
- 1/4 teaspoon paprika
- 1 teaspoon Celtic sea salt
- 1 pinch cinnamon
- Vegetable soup
- Diced tomatoes (canned)
- 2.3oz. of peas
- Preparation of cassava flour spoon

Directions:

1. Roughly cut vegetables and potatoes, then mash the garlic. Cut the pea sugar in half.
2. Place carrots, sweet potatoes and onions in a slow cooker.
3. Mix cassava flour with curry, cumin, chili, salt and cinnamon powder, and sprinkle with vegetables.
4. Pour the vegetable soup on top.
5. Close the lid of the slow cooker and cook on low heat for 6 hours.
6. Mix tomatoes and pea sugar in the last hour.
7. Cauliflower rice is an excellent addition to this dish.

Nutrition:

- Calories: 2395
- Sodium: 39 mg
- Dietary Fiber: 1.8 g
- Total Fat: 4.8 g
- Total Carbs: 16.7 g
- Protein: 1.4 g

74.   Buckwheat Toasted Muesli

Preparation time: 10 minutes

Cooking time: 30 minutes

Servings: 1

Ingredients:

- 4 cups of puffed buckwheat
- 2 cups of buckwheat flakes
- 3 cups of walnuts, chopped
- ½ cup of melted coconut oil
- 1/3 cup of honey
- 2 tablespoon cinnamon (ground)
- 2 tablespoon vanilla extract
- 1 teaspoon salt

Directions:

1. To complete this recipe, you will need to do the following:
2. Turn on the oven to 300 degrees Fahrenheit and preheat.
3. Combine your dry ingredients together and mix well.
4. In a pan, melt your coconut oil with your honey and vanilla. Wait for it to warm up to be runny, but do not let it boil or burn. It should just be runny.
5. Pour the liquid into the dry mixture and mix well until all ingredients are thoroughly coated
6. Spread out across the entire baking tray (lined with parchment paper)
7. Bake for 25 minutes, turning every 10 minutes to prevent burning
8. Remove from the oven and let it cool. It may not seem done at first, but be aware that it will crisp up when it is cool
9. When cool, move it to an airtight container. It should keep for about a month.

Nutrition:
- Calories: 267

- Sodium: 33 mg
- Dietary Fiber: 1.4 g
- Total Fat: 4.1 g
- Total Carbs: 16.7 g
- Protein: 1.6 g

75.   Eggs With Kale

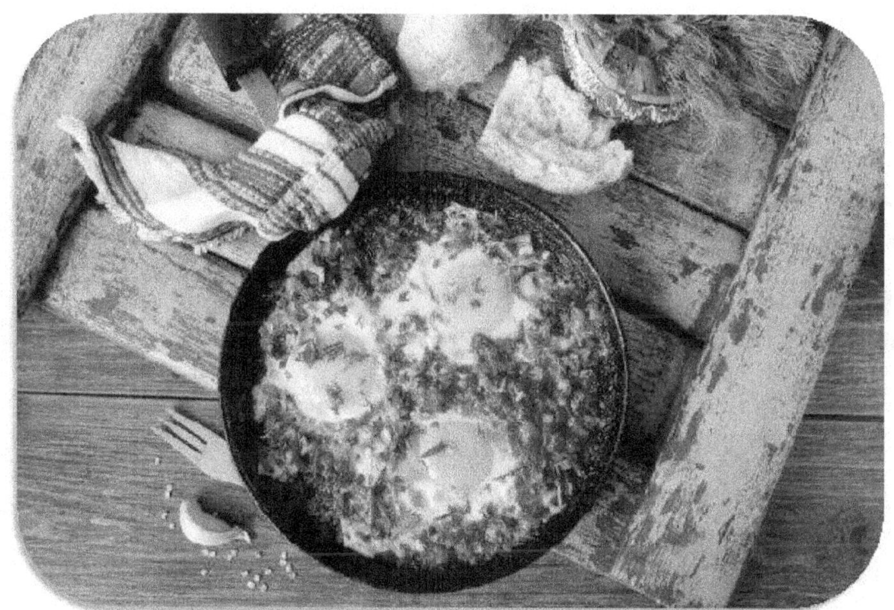

Preparation time: 15 minutes

Cooking time: 25 minutes

Total time: 40 minutes

Servings: 4

Ingredients:

- 2 tablespoons olive oil
- 1 yellow onion, chopped
- 2 garlic cloves, minced
- 1 cup tomatoes, chopped
- ½ pound fresh kale, tough ribs removed and chopped
- 1 teaspoon ground cumin
- ¼ teaspoon red pepper flakes, crushed
- Salt and ground black pepper, to taste
- 4 eggs

- 2 tablespoons fresh parsley, chopped

Directions:

1. Heat the oil in a large wok over medium heat and sauté the onion for about 4–5 minutes.
2. Add garlic and sauté for about 1 minute.
3. Add the tomatoes, spices, salt, and black pepper, and cook for about 2–3 minutes, stirring frequently.
4. Stir in the kale and cook for about 4–5 minutes.
5. Carefully, crack eggs on top of kale mixture.
6. With the lid, cover the wok and cook for about 10 minutes, or until desired doneness of eggs.
7. Serve hot with the garnishing of parsley.

Nutrition:

- Calories 175
- Sodium: 28 mg
- Dietary Fiber: 2.4 g
- Total Fat: 3.4 g
- Total Carbs: 14.3 g
- Protein: 1.3 g

76.   Green Egg Scramble

Preparation time: 10 minutes

Cooking time: 20 minutes

Servings: 1

Ingredients:

- 3 cups of kale and arugula, chopped and packed
- 4 eggs
- 1/8 cup of sliced green onions
- 2 teaspoons fresh tarragon (chopped)
- 1 tablespoon sour cream
- 1 tablespoon butter (unsalted)
- 1 tablespoon olive oil

Directions:

1. Add your oil to a skillet on medium-high heat and wait until shimmering. Then, add the arugula and kale and a pinch of salt. Cook and toss occasionally, until wilted, 4 minutes usually. Remove spinach and set aside.
2. Wipe out the skillet and return to burner
3. Add eggs, chives, tarragon, and a pinch of salt and pepper to a bowl and whisk until well combined and starting to bubble.
4. Melt butter into a skillet on medium-high heat and add egg mixture. Stir slowly with a spatula until eggs start to set (1 minute or so). Add in the greens and fold them into the eggs until softly set.
5. Remove from heat and add the sour cream, gently folding it in. Serve

Nutrition:

- Calories: 495
- Sodium: 32 mg
- Dietary Fiber: 1.7 g
- Total Fat: 4.2 g

- Total Carbs: 15.3 g
- Protein: 1.3 g

Chapter 6:   Soup Recipes

77.   Chicken, Kale and Lentil Soup

Preparation time: 10 minutes

Cooking time: 20 minutes

Servings: 1

Ingredients:

- 5 cups chicken or vegetable broth
- 1 minced chicken breast (good use for remaining chicken broths from other recipes!
- 1 small red onion
- 2 Cups of finely chopped kale
- 1 cup chopped spinach
- 1 cup lentils
- 1 celery stalk, chopped
- 1 carrot, chopped
- 1 little pepper or a pinch of cayenne pepper
- A pinch of salt
- 1 teaspoon extra virgin olive oil

Direction:

1. Cook the lentils according to the package, but take them out only a few minutes before they are cooked. Put aside.
2. Put the vegetables in a large saucepan and sauté in a little oil over medium heat. Stir until the vegetables are softer but not well cooked. Add the chicken (pre-cooked skinless chicken), add the reserved lentils, and cook for another 3 to 5 minutes. Add a pinch of salt.
3. Add the broth, simmer and simmer for 20 minutes. Stay away from heat. Serve as fresh.

Nutrition:

- Calories: 395
- Sodium: 31 mg
- Dietary Fiber: 1.5 g
- Total Fat: 3.1 g
- Total Carbs: 15.3 g
- Protein: 1.2 g

78.   Spicy Asian Noodle Soup

Preparation time: 10 minutes

Cooking time: 20 minutes

Servings: 1

Ingredients:

- 1 packet of buckwheat noodles, prepared as directed on the package
- 1 small red onion
- 2 Celery stalks, washed and chopped
- 1 piece of ginger, diced
- 1 garlic clove, chopped
- 1 cup arugula
- ¼ cup basil leaves, clean, dry, then chop
- ¼ cup walnuts
- 1 A teaspoon of sesame seeds
- 2 Tablespoons of black currant
- ½ chili
- 5 cups chicken or vegetable broth
- ½ lime juice
- One teaspoon extra virgin olive oil
- 1 tablespoon soya sauce

Direction:

1. Cook the pasta according to the instructions and set aside.
2. Sauté all the vegetables, ginger, garlic, chili and nuts in a pan over deficient heat for about 10 minutes. Add the broth and simmer for another 5 minutes.
3. Cut the pasta (roughly) so that it is small enough to be eaten comfortably in a soup.
4. Add this to the broth, add the sesame seeds and lime juice and remove from the heat.
5. Refrigerate and serve.

Nutrition:

- Calories: 495
- Sodium: 33 mg
- Dietary Fiber: 1.1 g
- Total Fat: 4.2 g
- Total Carbs: 16.3 g
- Protein: 1.4 g

79.   Shrimp and Arugula Soup

Preparation time: 10 minutes

Cooking time: 30 minutes

Servings: 2

Ingredients:

- 10 medium-sized shrimp or 5 large shrimp, clean, shelled and gutted
- 1 small red onion, thinly sliced
- 1 cup arugula
- 1 Kale
- 2 large celery stalks, thinly sliced
- 5 sprigs of chopped parsley
- 11 chopped garlic cloves
- 5 cups chicken or fish or vegetable broth
- 1 tablespoon. Extra virgin olive oil
- A pinch of sea salt
- A pinch of pepper

Direction:

1. Fry the vegetables (not yet kale or arugula) in a saucepan over low heat for about 2 minutes so that they are tender and crisp, but not yet cooked. You must save the cooking time for the next step. Add salt and pepper.
2. Then clean and cut the shrimp into small pieces that can be easily eaten in a soup. Then put the shrimp in the pan and sauté for another 10 minutes over medium heat. Make sure the shrimp is well cooked and not translucent.
3. When the shrimp seems well cooked, add the broth to the pan and cook over medium heat for about 20 minutes.
4. Remove from heat and let cool before serving.

Nutrition:

- Calories: 120,
- Sodium: 23 mg,
- Dietary Fiber: 2.4 g,
- Total Fat: 2.1 g,
- Total Carbs: 1.3 g,
- Protein: 10.3 g.

80.   Indian Lentil Soup

Preparation time: 10 minutes

Cooking time: 30 minutes

Servings: 2

Ingredients:

- 2 cups of lentils
- 1 small red onion, chopped
- 1 celery stalk, finely chopped
- 1 chopped carrot
- 2 large finely chopped kale leaves or 1 cup chopped kale
- 2 Coriander sprigs, chopped
- 3 Sprigs of chopped parsley
- ¼-1/2 hot pepper, seeded and chopped (use more or less as desired)
- 1 tomato, cut into small pieces
- 1 piece of ginger, chopped
- 1 garlic clove, chopped
- 5 cups chicken or vegetable broth
- 1 teaspoon of turmeric
- 1 teaspoon extra virgin olive oil ½ teaspoon salt

Direction:

1. Cook the lentils according to the package and remove them from the stove about 5 minutes before finishing.
2. Fry all the vegetables in olive oil in a pan. Then add the chopped vegetables at the end. Then add the ginger, garlic and chili and the turmeric powder.
3. Add the broth and simmer for 5 minutes. Add the lentils and salt.
4. Add the pre-cooked lentils and cook over low heat for another 25 minutes. Take it out of the stove and let it cool.
5. Cut the avocado, remove the hole and cut it, then remove the slices just before eating.

6. Cover with an avocado slice and serve immediately.

Nutrition:

- Calories: 120,
- Sodium: 23 mg,
- Dietary Fiber: 2.4 g,
- Total Fat: 2.1 g,
- Total Carbs: 1.3 g,
- Protein: 10.3 g.

81.   Broccoli And Kale Green Soup

Preparation time: 15 Minutes

Cooking time: 20 Minutes

Serving: 2

Ingredients:

- 1 tablespoon of sunflower oil
- 500ml, by mixing powder of 1 tablespoon broth and boiling water in a jug
- 2 garlic cloves, sliced
- Sliced ½ tsp of ground coriander, thumb-sized piece ginger.
- 1/2 teaspoon of fresh turmeric root, peeled and grated.
- Broccoli
- Kale, chopped
- Courgettes, roughly sliced
- One lime, zested and juiced
- A thin, finely chopped parsley pack with a few whole leaves.

Directions:

1. In a deep pot, place the butter, add the garlic, ginger, coriander, salt and turmeric, and fry over medium heat for 2 minutes, then add 3 tablespoons of water, and give the spices a little more moisture.
2. Add the courgettes, ensure that the slices have a good mixture of all the spices, then cook 3 minutes. Add stock of 400 ml and cook for 3 minutes.
3. Add the remaining stock to the broccoli, kale and lime juice. Let all vegetables soften and cook once more for 3-4 minutes.
4. Turn off the heat and add the pickled parsley. Load it all into a machine and blend it easily to high speed. It'll be a pretty leaf with patches of shadow (the kale). Decorate with parsley and lime.

Nutrition:

- Calories: 210,
- Sodium: 23 mg,
- Dietary Fiber: 6.4 g,
- Total Fat: 2.1 g,
- Total Carbs: 2.3 g,
- Protein: 10.3 g.

82.   Tofu & Shiitake Mushroom Soup

Preparation time: 10 minutes

Cooking time: 40 minutes

Servings: 1

Ingredient:

- 0.9oz dried wakame
- Vegetable stock
- 1.5oz shiitake mushrooms, sliced
- 2.5oz miso paste
- 14oz firm tofu, diced
- 2 green onion, trimmed and diagonally chopped
- 1 bird's eye chili, finely chopped

Direction:

1. Soak the wakame in lukewarm water for 10-15 minutes before draining.
2. In a medium-sized saucepan, add the vegetable stock and bring to the boil. Toss in the mushrooms and simmer for 2-3 minutes.
3. Mix miso paste with 3-4 tablespoon of vegetable stock from the saucepan until the miso is entirely dissolved. Pour the miso-stock back into the pan and add the tofu, wakame, green onions and chili, then serve immediately.

Nutrition:

- Calories: 295
- Sodium: 33 mg
- Dietary Fiber: 1.3 g
- Total Fat: 4.3 g
- Total Carbs: 16.3 g
- Protein: 1.2 g

83.   Overnight Buckwheat Porridge

Preparation time: 10 minutes

Cooking time: 20 minutes

Servings: 1

Ingredients:

- 1 cup of buckwheat groats
- ¼ cup of chia seeds
- 3 cups of soy milk (you can sub this for any of the milk that you choose, cow's or otherwise)
- 1 cup of water
- A pinch of cinnamon
- A pinch of salt
- 2 teaspoons vanilla
- ½ cup crushed unsalted walnuts
- 1.5 cups chopped strawberries and blueberries

Directions:

1. This recipe is incredibly simple to start the night before all you have to do is the following:
2. Mix everything but the berries and nuts in a bowl, seal it, and leave in the fridge overnight.
3. When you are ready to eat it, pull it out, add it to a pot, and stir for 10-12 minutes over medium heat until it is the desired texture.
4. Add the fruits and nuts and serve.

Nutrition:

- Calories: 1495
- Sodium: 23 mg
- Dietary Fiber: 1.5 g
- Total Fat: 3.1 g
- Total Carbs: 16.7 g
- Protein: 1.8 g

84.   Buckwheat Porridge

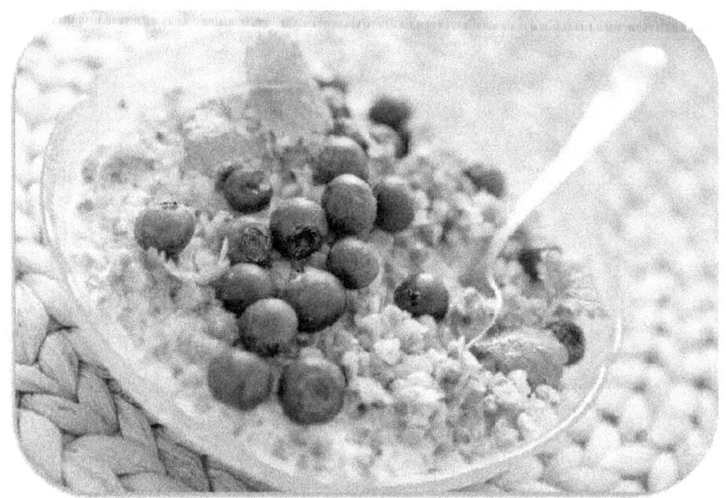

Preparation time: 10 minutes

Cooking time: 15 minutes

Total time: 25 minutes

Servings: 2

Ingredients:

- 1 cup buckwheat, rinsed
- 1 cup unsweetened almond milk
- 1 cup water
- ½ teaspoon ground cinnamon
- ½ teaspoon vanilla extract
- 1–2 tablespoons raw honey
- ¼ cup fresh blueberries

Directions:

1. In a pan, add all the ingredients (except honey and blueberries) over medium-high heat and bring to a boil.
2. Now, reduce the heat to low and simmer, covered for about 10 minutes.
3. Stir in the honey and remove from the heat.
4. Set aside, covered, for about 5 minutes.
5. With a fork, fluff the mixture, and transfer into serving bowls.
6. Top with blueberries and serve.

Nutrition:

- Calories: 358
- Sodium: 38 mg,
- Dietary Fiber: 2.2 g,
- Total Fat: 5.1 g,
- Total Carbs: 16.4 g,
- Protein: 1.7 g.

85.   Date and Walnut Porridge

Preparation Time: 10 minutes

Cooking time: 0 minute

Servings: 1

Ingredients:

- 200 ml Milk or dairy-free alternative
- 1 teaspoon. Walnut butter or four chopped walnut halves
- 1 Medjool date, chopped
- 1.75 ounces of Strawberries, hulled
- 1.45 ounces of Buckwheat flakes

Directions:

1. Place the milk and date in a saucepan, heat gently, then add the buckwheat flakes and cook until the porridge is the consistency you like.
2. Stir in the butter of walnut or walnuts, top with the strawberries and serve.

Nutrition:

- Calories 183
- Sodium: 26 mg
- Dietary Fiber: 2.8 g
- Total Fat: 2.1 g
- Total Carbs: 14.3 g
- Protein: 1.2 g

Chapter 7:   Salads Recipes

86.   Smoked Salmon Salad

Preparation time: 10 minutes

Cooking time: 0 minutes

Servings: 1

Ingredients:

- 1 cup or ¼ packet (if significant) of smoked salmon slices (no cooking required!)
- 1 avocado, seeded, sliced and picked
- 10 chopped nuts
- 5 wild celery (or celery leaves), chopped
- 2 celery sticks, finely chopped or sliced
- ½ small red onion, thinly sliced
- 1 boneless Medjool date, chopped
- 1 tablespoon. Capers
- 1 tablespoon. Extra virgin olive oil
- 1/4 lemon, squeezed
- 5 sprigs of chopped parsley

Direction:

1. Wash and dry salads and vegetables, cover with salmon.

Nutrition:

- Calories: 95
- Sodium: 22 mg
- Dietary Fiber: 1.6 g
- Total Fat: 3.1 g
- Total Carbs: 1.3 g
- Protein: 1.3 g

87.   Lentil Salad

Preparation time: 10 minutes

Cooking time: 0 minutes

Servings: 1

Ingredients:

- 1 cup cooked red lentils (prepared, hot or used at room temperature)
- 1 Avocado, pitted, sliced and removed
- 2 Cups of chopped kale
- 2 celery sticks, finely chopped or sliced
- ½ small red onion, thinly sliced
- 1 boneless Medjool date, chopped
- ¼ cup red currants
- 1 teaspoon of turmeric
- 1 tablespoon. Extra virgin olive oil
- 1/4 lemon, squeezed
- 5 sprigs of chopped parsley

Direction:

1. Add the ingredients and mix gently. To serve

Nutrition:

- Calories: 195,
- Sodium: 30 mg,
- Dietary Fiber: 1.4 g,
- Total Fat: 4.0 g,
- Total Carbs: 16.2 g,
- Protein: 1.5 g.

88.   Tomato Cream With Crunchy Capers

Preparation time: 10 Minutes,

Cooking time: 30 Minutes,

Servings: 4

Ingredients:

- 2 tablespoons of triple tomato paste
- 1 clove of garlic
- 1 onion dried oregano
- Lemon peel
- Salt
- Pepper
- 4 tablespoons of salted capers
- 4 spoons of extra virgin olive oil
- Tomato pulp

Directions:

1. In a saucepan, brown the onion and garlic in olive oil, add the triple tomato paste and the pulp. Season with salt and cook until you get a thick cream. In a small pan, heat the oil, dip the desalted capers and leave them on the fire until they become crispy.
2. Collect them, dry them on kitchen paper. Transfer the tomato cream to four small single-serving cocottas, add the crunchy capers, oregano, and lemon zest to taste. Complete with a round of extra virgin olive oil and a mince of fresh reel pepper. Serve immediately.

Nutrition:

- Calories: 270
- Sodium: 13 mg
- Dietary Fiber: 6.4 g
- Total Fat: 3.1 g
- Total Carbs: 213 g
- Protein: 10.3 g

89.   Kale & Raspberry Salad

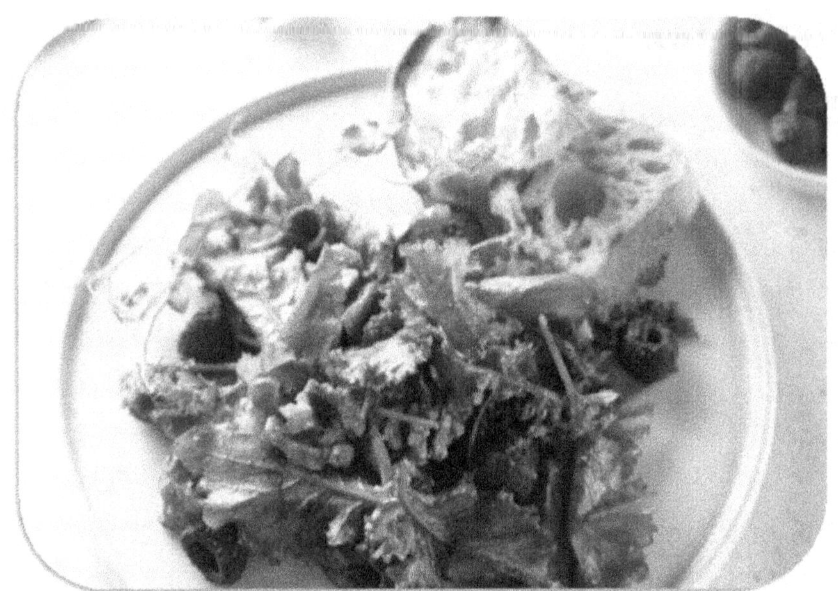

Preparation time: 15 minutes

Cooking time: 15 minutes

Servings: 2

Ingredients:

- 3 cups fresh baby kale
- ½ cup fresh raspberries
- ¼ cup walnuts, chopped

Dressing:

- 1 tablespoon extra-virgin olive oil
- 1 tablespoon apple cider vinegar
- ½ teaspoon pure maple syrup
- Salt and ground black pepper, to taste

Directions:

1. For salad: in a salad bowl, place all ingredients and mix.

2. For the dressing: place all ingredients in another bowl and beat until well combined.
3. Place dressing on top of the salad and toss to coat well.
4. Serve immediately.

Nutrition:

- Calories: 270,
- Sodium: 13 mg,
- Dietary Fiber: 6.4 g,
- Total Fat: 3.1 g,
- Total Carbs: 213 g,
- Protein: 10.3 g.

90.   Kale & Citrus Fruit Salad

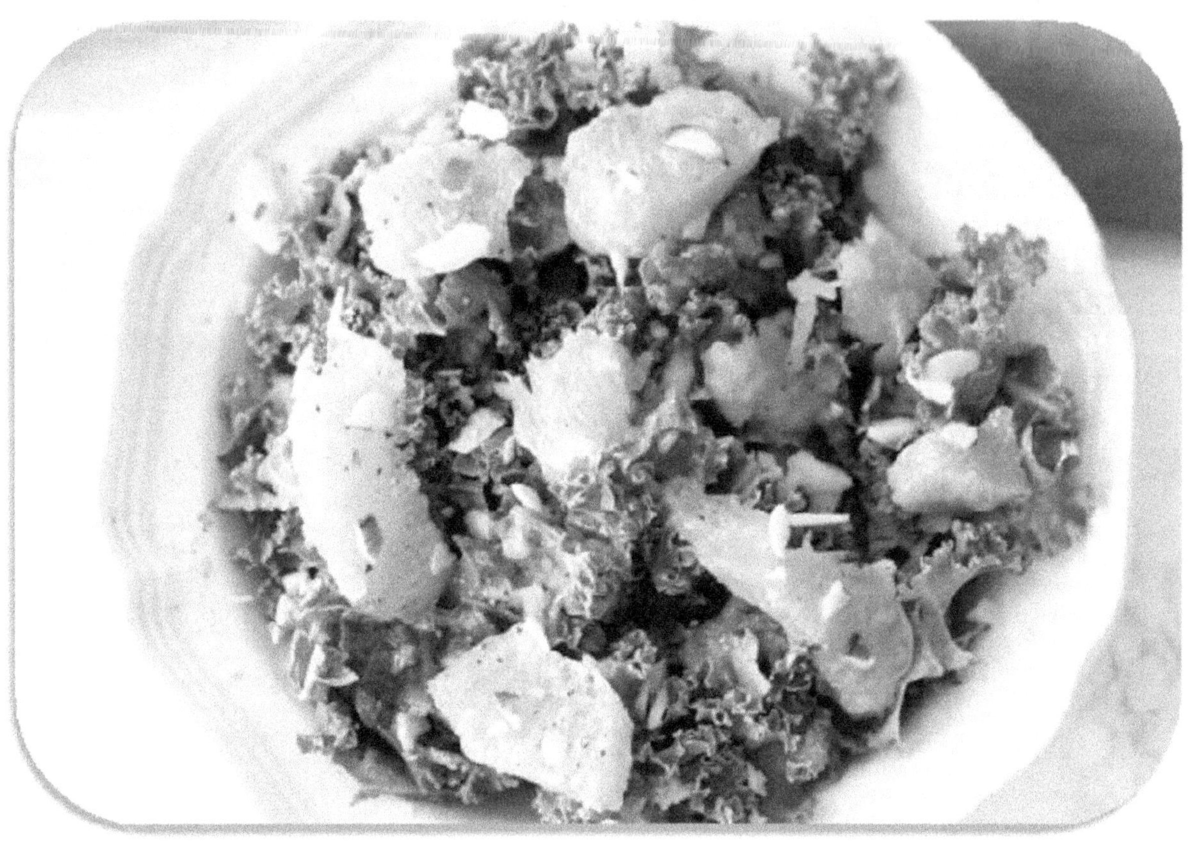

Preparation time: 15 minutes

Total time: 15 minutes

Servings: 2

Ingredients:

- 3 cups fresh kale, tough ribs removed and torn
- 1 orange, peeled and segmented
- 1 grapefruit, peeled and segmented
- 2 tablespoons unsweetened dried cranberries
- ¼ teaspoon white sesame seeds

Dressing:

- 2 tablespoons extra-virgin olive oil
- 2 tablespoons fresh orange juice
- 1 teaspoon Dijon mustard
- ½ teaspoon raw honey
- Salt and ground black pepper, to taste

Directions

1. For salad: in a salad bowl, place all ingredients and mix.
2. For the dressing: place all ingredients in another bowl and beat until well combined.
3. Place dressing on top of the salad and toss to coat well.
4. Serve immediately.

Nutrition:

- Calories: 270
- Sodium: 13 mg
- Dietary Fiber: 6.4 g
- Total Fat: 3.1 g
- Total Carbs: 213 g
- Protein: 10.3 g

91. Arugula & Berries Salad

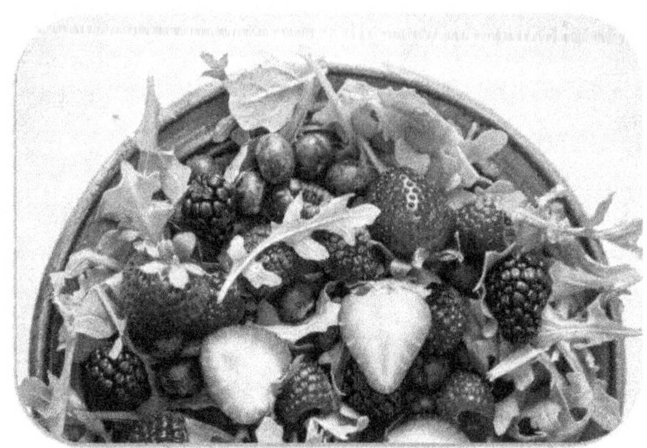

Preparation time: 15 minutes

Cooking time: 0 minutes

Servings: 4

Ingredients:

- 1 cup fresh strawberries, hulled and sliced
- ½ cup fresh blackberries
- ½ cup fresh blueberries
- ½ cup fresh raspberries
- 6 cups fresh arugula
- 2 tablespoons extra-virgin olive oil
- Salt and ground black pepper, to taste

Directions:

1. In a salad bowl, place all the ingredients and toss to coat well.
2. Serve immediately.

Nutrition:

- Calories: 270
- Sodium: 13 mg

- Dietary Fiber: 6.4 g
- Total Fat: 3.1 g
- Total Carbs: 213 g
- Protein: 10.3 g

92.   Baked Salmon Salad With Creamy Mint Dressing

Preparation Time: 20 minutes

Cooking time: 20 minutes

Servings: 1

Ingredients:

- 1 salmon fillet (130g)
- Mixed salad leaves
- 2 radishes, trimmed and thinly sliced
- 1.76 ounces of young spinach leaves
- 5cm piece cucumber, cut into chunks
- 1 small handful (10g) parsley, roughly chopped
- 2 spring onions, trimmed and sliced
- For the dressing:
- 1 tablespoon natural yogurt
- 1 teaspoon low-fat mayonnaise
- 2 leaves mint, finely chopped
- 1 tablespoon rice vinegar
- Salt and freshly ground black pepper

Directions:

1. Firstly, you heat the oven to 200 ° C (180 ° C fan / Gas 6).
2. Place the salmon filet on a baking tray and bake for 16– 18 minutes until you have just cooked. Remove, and set aside from the oven. The salmon in the salad is equally nice and hot or cold. If your salmon has skin, cook the skin side down and remove the salmon from the skin after cooking, use a slice of fish. When cooked, it should slide away easily.
3. Mix the mayonnaise, yogurt, rice wine vinegar, mint leaves and salt and pepper in a small dish and let it stand for at least 5 minutes for aromas to evolve.

4. Place on a serving plate the salad leaves and spinach, and top with the radishes, the cucumber, the spring onions and the parsley. Flake the cooked salmon over the salad and sprinkle over the dressing.

Nutrition:

- Calories: 270
- Sodium: 13 mg
- Dietary Fiber: 6.4 g
- Total Fat: 3.1 g
- Total Carbs: 213 g
- Protein: 10.3 g

93.   Sirt Fruit Salad

Preparation time: 10 minutes

Cooking time: 20 minutes

Servings: 2

Ingredients:

- 1 cup freshly made green tea
- 1 fresh orange juice
- 1 orange, chopped
- 2 green apples, cored and roughly chopped
- 20 red seedless grapes
- 10 blueberries
- 2 teaspoon honey

Directions:

1. Stir the honey into a cup of green tea. When dissolved, add the orange juice. Leave to cool.
2. Place the chopped orange, chopped apple, grapes, and blueberries together in a bowl. Pour the cool green tea over it and leave to steep for some minutes before serving.

Nutrition:

- Calories: 270
- Sodium: 13 mg
- Dietary Fiber: 6.4 g
- Total Fat: 3.1 g
- Total Carbs: 213 g
- Protein: 10.3 g

94.   Greek Salad Skewers

Preparation time: 10 minutes

Cooking time: 0 minute

Servings: 1

Ingredients:

- 2 wooden skewers, soaked in water for 30 minutes before use
- 8 large black olives
- 8 cherry tomatoes
- 1 yellow pepper, cut into eight squares
- ½ red onion, chopped in half and separated into eight pieces
- 3.5-ounces (about 10cm) cucumber, cut into four slices and halved
- 3.5 ounces of feta, cut into eight cubes
- For the dressing:
- 1 tablespoon extra-virgin olive oil
- 1 teaspoon balsamic vinegar
- Juice of ½ lemon
- Few leaves basil, finely chopped (or ½ tsp dried mixed herbs to replace basil and oregano)
- A right amount of salt and freshly ground black pepper
- Few leaves oregano, finely chopped
- ½ clove garlic, peeled and crushed

Directions:

1. Thread each skewer in the order with salad ingredients: olive, tomato, yellow pepper, red onion, cucumber, feta, basil, olive, yellow pepper, red ointment, cucumber, feta.
2. Put all the ingredients of the dressing in a small bowl and blend well together. Pour over the spoils.

Nutrition:

- Calories: 270

- Sodium: 13 mg
- Dietary Fiber: 6.4 g
- Total Fat: 3.1 g
- Total Carbs: 213 g
- Protein: 10.3 g

95.   Salmon Salad

Preparation time: 10 minutes

Cooking time: 10 minutes

Servings: 1

Ingredients:

- 3 cups of arugula
- 3 cups of chicory leaves
- ½ cup sliced smoked salmon
- ½ of an avocado, peeled and sliced
- 6 walnuts, crushed,
- 1 tablespoon capers
- 1 large Medjool date, pitted and chopped
- 1 tablespoon of olive oil
- ¼ lemon, juiced
- 10 sprigs of parsley, chopped
- 1 medium stalk of celery, chopped
- ½ cup thinly sliced red onion

Directions:

1. Chop and prepare all ingredients
2. Place salad leaves into a large bowl
3. Mix the remaining ingredients together in another bowl and pour on top of the leaves. Serve

Nutrition:

- Calories: 270
- Sodium: 13 mg
- Dietary Fiber: 6.4 g
- Total Fat: 3.1 g
- Total Carbs: 213 g
- Protein: 10.3 g

96.   Melon and Ham Salad

Preparation time: 10 minutes

Cooking time: 10 minutes

Servings: 2

Ingredients:

- Arugula
- 8 slices of Serrano ham
- Rocket
- Cucumber (cut into thin slices)
- 1 slice of red onion (ring)

Directions:

1. In 3 tablespoons of olive oil, prepare a quarter of melon. Use a spoon to remove, cut and peel. Then cut the melon into equal parts.
2. Cut the ham into thin slices.
3. Put arugula, cucumber and onion in a bowl.
4. Sprinkle olive oil on the salad.
5. Spread it on a plate, then place a part of the melon on it.

Nutrition:

- Calories: 270
- Sodium: 13 mg
- Dietary Fiber: 6.4 g
- Total Fat: 3.1 g
- Total Carbs: 213 g
- Protein: 10.3 g

97. Coronation Chicken Salad

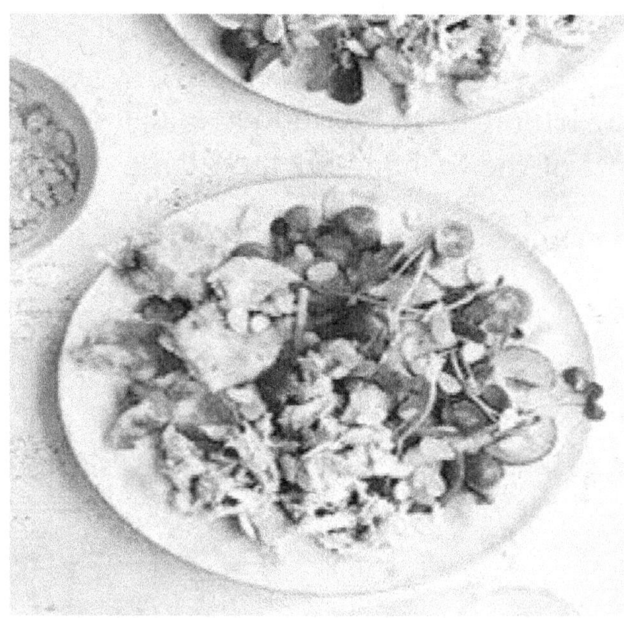

Preparation time: 10 minutes

Cooking time: 45 minutes

Servings: 2

Ingredients:

- 1.4 ounces of Natural yogurt
- Juice of 1/4 of a lemon
- 1 teaspoon Coriander, hacked
- 1 teaspoon ground turmeric
- 1/2 teaspoon Mild curry powder
- 3 ounces of cooked chicken bosom, cut into scaled-down pieces
- 6 Walnut parts, finely hacked
- 1 Medjool date, finely hacked
- 1 ounce of Red onion, diced
- 1 Bird's eye stew

- 1.2 ounces of Rocket, to serve

Directions:

1. Blend the yogurt, lemon juice, coriander and flavors together in a bowl. Include all the rest of the fixings and serve on a bed of the rocket.

Nutrition:

- Calories: 270
- Sodium: 13 mg
- Dietary Fiber: 6.4 g
- Total Fat: 3.1 g
- Total Carbs: 213 g
- Protein: 10.3 g

98.   Mung Beans Snack Salad

Preparation time: 10 minutes

Cooking time: 0 minutes

Servings: 6

Ingredients:

- 2 cups tomatoes, chopped
- 2 cups cucumber, chopped
- 3 cups mixed greens
- 2 cups mung beans, sprouted
- 2 cups clover sprouts
- For the salad dressing:
- 1 tablespoon cumin, ground
- 1 cup dill, chopped
- 4 tablespoons lemon juice
- 1 avocado, pitted, peeled and roughly chopped
- 1 cucumber, roughly chopped

Directions:

1. In a salad bowl, mix tomatoes with 2 cups cucumber, greens, clover and mung sprouts.
2. In your blender, mix cumin with dill, lemon juice, 1 cucumber and avocado, blend really well, add this to your salad, toss well and serve as a snack

Enjoy!

Nutrition:

- Calories: 210
- Sodium: 13 mg
- Dietary Fiber: 6.4 g
- Total Fat: 3.1 g
- Total Carbs: 213 g

- Protein: 2.3 g

99.   Sirt Super Salad

Preparation time: 20 minutes

Cooking time: 0 minutes

Servings: 1

Ingredients:

- 1 3/4 ounces of endive leaves
- 1 3/4 ounces of arugula
- 3 1/2 ounces of smoked salmon slices
- 1/2 cup of celery, including leaves, sliced
- 1/2 cup of avocado, peeled, stoned, and sliced
- 1/8 cups of walnuts, chopped
- 1/8 cup of red onion, sliced
- One tablespoon of capers
- One tablespoon of extra virgin olive oil
- One large Medjool date, pitted and chopped
- Juice of 1/4 lemon
- 1/4 cup of parsley, chopped

Directions:

1. On a plate or wide cup, place the salad leaves.
2. Mix all the remaining ingredients and pour over the seeds.

Nutrition:

- Calories: 210
- Sodium: 13 mg
- Dietary Fiber: 6.4 g
- Total Fat: 3.1 g
- Total Carbs: 213 g
- Protein: 2.3 g

100.   Sprouts and Apples Snack Salad

Preparation time: 10 minutes

Cooking time: 0 minutes

Servings: 4

Ingredients:

- 1-pound Brussels sprouts, shredded
- 1 cup walnuts, chopped
- 1 apple, cored and cubed
- 1 red onion, chopped

For the salad dressing:

- 3 tablespoons red vinegar
- 1 tablespoon mustard
- ½ cup olive oil
- 1 garlic clove, minced
- Black pepper to the taste

Directions:

1. In a salad bowl, mix sprouts with apple, onion and walnuts.
2. In another bowl, mix vinegar with mustard, oil, garlic and pepper, whisk really well, add this to your salad, toss well and serve as a snack.

Enjoy!

Nutrition:

- Calories: 210
- Sodium: 13 mg
- Dietary Fiber: 6.4 g
- Total Fat: 3.1 g
- Total Carbs: 213 g
- Protein: 2.3 g

101. Chicken Sirtfood Salad

Preparation time: 10 minutes

Cooking time: 10 minutes

Servings: 1

Ingredients:

- ¼ cup plain Greek yogurt
- ¼ lemon, juiced
- 1 teaspoon conciliator, finely chopped
- 1 teaspoon turmeric powder
- ½ teaspoon curry powder (more to taste if you prefer it spicy)
- ¾ cup cooked chicken breast into bite-sized pieces
- 3 whole walnuts, crushed
- 1 Medjool date, pitted and diced
- 1/8 cup diced red onion
- 1 bird's eye chili, diced (remove seeds if you do not want it to be too spicy)
- 2.5 cups roughly chopped arugula

Directions:

To make this recipe, you will need to do the following:

1. In a medium-sized bowl, combine your Greek yogurt, the juice from the lemon, your cilantro, and the curry and turmeric powders. Combine well.
2. Add in your chicken, walnuts, date, onion, and chili and mix together thoroughly.
3. Add to the top of the arugula. Serve.

Nutrition:

- Calories: 210
- Sodium: 13 mg
- Dietary Fiber: 6.4 g
- Total Fat: 3.1 g
- Total Carbs: 213 g

- Protein: 2.3 g

102.   Sirtfood Pesto Buckwheat Salad

Preparation time: 10 minutes

Cooking time: 10 minutes

Servings: 1

Ingredients:

- 4 cups of parsley
- 1 teaspoon minced garlic
- 1 lemon, juiced
- ½ cup of walnuts
- 3 bird's eye chilis remove the seeds if you do not like spicy food
- ½ cup cauliflower, broken down
- 2 tablespoon parmesan cheese, freshly shredded
- 2 tablespoons extra-virgin olive oil
- 2 tablespoons water
- Salt and pepper to taste
- 2 cups diced chicken breast, cooked
- 8 oz buckwheat pasta (dry weight), cooked

Directions:

To complete this recipe, you will need to do the following:

1. Prepare your chicken and pasta, and set aside in a large bowl.
2. In a food processor, combine all ingredients aside from chicken and pasta. Blend until the consistency of pesto. Stop and scrape down walls from time to time to mix well.
3. Add 1 cup of pesto to the pasta and mix. If still dry, add more pesto to taste and mix well.
4. Store in the fridge until ready to eat.

Nutrition:

- Calories: 210
- Sodium: 13 mg
- Dietary Fiber: 6.4 g
- Total Fat: 3.1 g
- Total Carbs: 213 g
- Protein: 2.3 g

103.   Red Chicory, Pear and Hazelnut Salad

Preparation time: 5 Minutes

Cooking time: 0 minutes

Serving: 1

Ingredients:

For the dressing:

- 1 teaspoon of sherry or cider vinegar
- Two heads of red chicory or white if not available
- 25g of hazelnuts, toasted and chopped
- Two ripe red Williams's pears
- A good handful of rocket leaves
- 2 tablespoons of hazelnut or olive oil
- 1 teaspoon of green peppercorns in brine, optional
- 2 tablespoons of salad oil, either sunflower oil or safflower oil.

Directions

1. Dress up. If using green peppercorn, lightly crush them in a bowl or use a pestle and mortar with a wooden spoon. Mix the oils and vinegar and sprinkle with the salt.
2. Remove the stalk from the chicory and any tired-looking external leaves.
3. Take the tongs out of the pears, and lengthwise quarter the pears. Cut the kernel and dice the fruit thinly. Arrange the chicory slices and spoon more than half of the sauce.
4. Pour the remaining dressing, salt and pepper seasoning over the rocket leaves.
5. Place the leaves on top of each salad and easily flip. Sprinkle and top with almonds.

Nutrition:

- Calories: 210
- Sodium: 13 mg

- Dietary Fiber: 6.4 g
- Total Fat: 3.1 g
- Total Carbs: 213 g
- Protein: 2.3 g

104.   Apple and Egg Salad

Preparation time: 10 minutes

Cooking time: 20 minutes

Servings: 1

Ingredients:

- Egg
- Apple (cubic)
- 1/2 chopped onion (chopped).
- 1/2 cucumber (cubic)

Directions:

1. Boil the eggs vigorously for 8 minutes, startle them, and then peel them in cold water.
2. Place lettuce, cucumbers, onions and apples in a large bowl.
3. Cut the eggs into small pieces and put them in a bowl.
4. Season the salad with olive oil and season with salt and pepper.

Nutrition:

- Calories: 210
- Sodium: 13 mg
- Dietary Fiber: 6.4 g
- Total Fat: 3.1 g
- Total Carbs: 213 g
- Protein: 2.3 g

105.   Sweet Potato Salad With Bacon

Preparation time: 10 minutes

Cooking time: 30 minutes

Servings: 1

Ingredients:

- Five slices of bacon
- Sweet potato (peeled and diced)
- Garlic clove (squeezed)
- A spoonful of lemon juice
- A spoon of olive oil
- Balsamic vinegar preparation spoon

Directions:

1. Preheat the oven to 220 ° C and cover the pan with parchment paper.
2. Place the bacon on the baking sheet and cook until crispy (about 20 minutes).
3. Remove the bacon from the pan, crisp and mince.
4. Mix the sweet potato cubes with garlic in the same pot, season with a little olive oil, and fry in the oven for about 30 minutes.
5. Seasoned olive oil, vinegar and lime juice in a bowl.
6. Remove the French fries from the oven, mix with bacon, French fries, and season with spices.
7. If necessary, add rockets and pine nuts at the end.

Nutrition:

- Calories: 210,
- Sodium: 13 mg,
- Dietary Fiber: 6.4 g,
- Total Fat: 3.1 g,
- Total Carbs: 213 g,
- Protein: 2.3 g.

106.   Italian Kale Salad

Preparation time 5 Minutes,

Cooking time: 5 Minutes

Servings: 8

This vibrant green dish was tasted and dressed in vinegar, giving it a sweet and sour taste, which keeps you coming back for more.

Ingredients:

- 3 tablespoons of red wine vinegar
- 3 garlic cloves, finely sliced
- 3 tablespoons of olive oil
- Cavolo Nero or kale, roughly shredded

Direction:

1. Then apply the vinegar and a splash of water to heat the oil into a large bowl with a plate, fill it with the garlic.
2. Top up the kale and cover the steam, adding more water if the pot gets too dry for 4-5 minutes. Season with a little sea salt once the kale gets wilted.

Nutrition:

- Calories: 104
- Sodium: 33 mg
- Dietary Fiber: 1.4 g
- Total Fat: 4.1 g
- Total Carbs: 16.3 g
- Protein: 1.3 g

107.   Avocado Salad Buffet

Preparation time: 10 minutes

Cooking time: 10 minutes

Servings: 2

Ingredients:

- 1/2 slices of cucumber
- 1 slice avocado
- 1 / 2 slices red onion
- 250g cold salad
- Smoked salmon steak:
- Cucumber, avocado and onion nuts.

Directions:

1. Spread lettuce leaves on a deep plate, then spread cucumber, avocado and onion on the salad.
2. Season with salt and pepper (you can also add olive oil to the salad).
3. Put the smoked salmon slices on it, then eat immediately.

Nutrition:

- Calories: 104
- Sodium: 113 mg
- Dietary Fiber: 0.4 g
- Total Fat: 4.1 g
- Total Carbs: 16.3 g
- Protein: 1.3 g

108.   Salmon and Shrimp Salad

Preparation time: 5 minutes

Cooking time: 0 minutes

Servings: 4

Ingredients:

- 1 cup smoked salmon, boneless and flaked
- 1 cup shrimp, peeled, deveined and cooked
- ½ cup baby arugula
- 1 tablespoon lemon juice
- 2 spring onions, chopped
- 1 tablespoon olive oil
- A pinch of sea salt and black pepper

Directions:

In a salad bowl, combine the salmon with the shrimp and the other ingredients, toss and serve.

Nutrition:

- Calories: 210
- Fat: 6g
- Fiber: 5g
- Carbs: 10g
- Protein: 12g

109.   Shrimp, Tomato and Dates Salad

Preparation time: 10 minutes

Cooking time: 0 mlnutes

Servings: 4

Ingredients:

- 1 pound shrimp, cooked, peeled and deveined
- 2 cups baby spinach
- 2 tablespoons walnuts, chopped
- 1 cup cherry tomatoes, halved
- 1 tablespoon lemon juice
- ½ cup dates, chopped
- 2 tablespoons avocado oil

Directions:

In a salad bowl, mix the shrimp with the spinach, walnuts and the other ingredients, toss and serve.

Nutrition:

- Calories: 243
- Fat: 5.4g
- Fiber: 3.3g
- Carbs: 21.6g
- Protein: 28.3g

110.   Salmon and Watercress Salad

Preparation time: 10 minutes

Cooking time: 0 minutes

Servings: 4

Ingredients:

- 1 pound smoked salmon, boneless, skinless and flaked
- 2 spring onions, chopped
- 2 tablespoons avocado oil
- ½ cup baby arugula
- 1 cup watercress
- 1 tablespoon lemon juice
- 1 cucumber, sliced
- 1 avocado, peeled, pitted and roughly cubed
- A pinch of sea salt and black pepper

Directions:

In a salad bowl, mix the salmon with the spring onions, watercress and the other ingredients, toss and serve.

Nutrition:

- Calories: 261
- Fat: 15.8g
- Fiber: 4.4g
- Carbs: 8.2g
- Protein: 22.7g

111. Salmon Salad with Creamy Dressing

Preparation Time: 12 minutes

Cooking Time: 10 minutes

Servings: 3

Ingredients:

- One salmon filet (130g)
- 40g blended plate of mixed greens leaves
- 40g youthful spinach leaves
- 40g youthful spinach leaves
- Two radishes, cut and daintily cut
- 5cm piece (50g) cucumber, cut into lumps
- Two spring onions, trimmed and cut
- One little bunch (10g) parsley, generally cleaved

Directions:

Place the salmon filet on a heating plate and prepare for 16–18 minutes until simply cooked through. Expel from the stove and put in a safe spot. The salmon is similarly pleasant hot or cold in the plate of mixed greens. On the off chance that your salmon has skin, cook skin side down and expel the salmon from the surface utilizing a fish cut after cooking. It should slide off effectively when cooked.

In a little bowl, combine the mayonnaise, yoghurt, rice wine vinegar, minutest leaves and salt and pepper and leave to represent in any event 5 minutes to permit the flavors to create.

Arrange the plate of mixed greens leaves and spinach on a serving plate and top with the radishes, cucumber, spring onions and parsley. Piece the cooked salmon onto the serving of mixed greens and shower the dressing over.

Nutrition:

- 13 calories

- 10 g complete fat
- 1.2 g immersed fat
- 31 mg cholesterol
- 20 mg sodium
- 83 mg potassium
- 2g starches
- 79 mcg folate
- 19 mg calcium

112. Strawberry, Tomato And Potato Salad With Honey & Pink Pepper Dressing

Preparation time: 10 Minutes,

Cooking time: 20 Minutes,

Servings: 4

Ingredients:

- Potatoes
- Strawberries
- Three tablespoon of extra virgin olive oil
- Two strawberries chopped
- For the dressing:
- Three tablespoons of pink peppercorns
- ½ lemon, juiced
- ½ tablespoon of honey
- Tomatoes

Directions

Toast the potatoes with a dry pot for 1-2 minutes, then cook quickly with a stick and a touch of Salt to split up the skins.

To prepare the sauce. Attach and crush the two strawberries into a paste.

Stir in the lemon juice and the honey. In a large bowl, put the dressing and the olive oil whisk. Please check the seasoning and if you like add a bit more salt or lemon juice. To assemble the bowl, split the strawberries into quarters or thin wedges, and finely slice the tomatoes, chopping some and halving others, so you get plenty of various shapes. In the bowl, mix with the hammer.

Place the salad on a tray to serve

Nutrition:

- Calories: 210,

- Sodium: 23 mg,
- Dietary Fibre: 6.4 g,
- Total Fat: 2.1 g,
- Total Carbs: 2.3 g,
- Protein: 10.3 g.

Chapter 8:   Omelettes Recipes

113.   Green Omelette

Preparation time: 10 minutes

Cooking time: 0 minute

Serves: 1

Ingredients:

- 1 tsp olive oil
- Two large eggs, at room temperature
- 1 shallot, peeled and finely chopped
- Small handful (10g) parsley, finely chopped
- Handful (20g) rocket leaves
- Salt and freshly ground black pepper

Directions:

1. In a frying pan heat, the oil at a medium to low heat and fry the shallot gently for 5 minutes. Switch the flame up a bit and then cook for another 2 minutes.
2. Whisk the eggs well in a bowl or cup along with a fork. Distribute the shallot around the pan equally before pouring the eggs in. Tip the pan slightly on either side to ensure an equal distribution of the egg.
3. Cook for about a minute before you raise the sides of the omelet. Then allow any runny egg to slip into the base of the pan. Sprinkle leaves and parsley immediately over the shot, and season generously with salt and pepper.
4. The top side of the omelet will still be soft but not runny when cooked, and the base will start browning. Spoon onto a plate and instantly enjoy.

Nutrition:

- Calories: 234
- Sodium: 33 mg,
- Dietary Fiber: 1.4 g,
- Total Fat: 4.4 g,
- Total Carbs: 16.7 g,
- Protein: 1.2 g.

114. Salmon & Kale Omelet

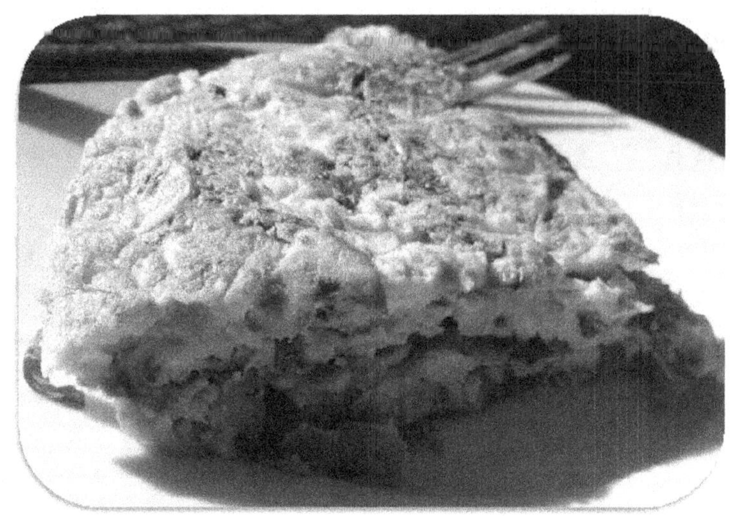

Preparation time: 10 minutes

Cooking time: 7 minutes

Total time: 17 minutes

Servings: 4

Ingredients:

- 6 eggs
- 2 tablespoons unsweetened almond milk
- Salt and ground black pepper, to taste
- 2 tablespoons olive oil
- 4 ounces smoked salmon, cut into bite-sized chunks
- 2 cup fresh kale, tough ribs removed and chopped finely
- 4 scallions, chopped finely

Directions:

1. In a bowl, place the eggs, coconut milk, salt, and black pepper, and beat well. Set aside.

2. In a non-stick wok, heat the oil over medium heat.
3. Place the egg mixture evenly and cook for about 30 seconds without stirring.
4. Place the salmon kale and scallions on top of the egg mixture evenly.
5. Now, reduce heat to low.
6. With the lid, cover the wok and cook for about 4–5 minutes, or until omelet is done completely.
7. Uncover the wok and cook for about 1 minute.
8. Carefully transfer the omelet onto a serving plate and serve.

Nutrition

- Calories 210
- Sodium: 31 mg
- Dietary Fiber: 1.4 g
- Total Fat: 4.2 g
- Total Carbs: 16.6 g
- Protein: 1.4 g

115.   Smoked Salmon Omelette

Preparation time: 10 minutes

Cooking time: 20 minutes

Servings: 2

Ingredients:

- 4 medium-size eggs
- 4 ounces of smoked salmon, sliced
- 1 teaspoon Capers
- 1 ounce of arugula (Rocket), chopped
- 2 teaspoon chopped parsley
- 2 teaspoon extra virgin olive oil.

Directions:

1. Crack eggs into a bowl and beat very well.
2. Add the salmon, rocket, capers, and parsley.
3. Heat the olive oil in a non-stick frying pan until hot but not smoking.
4. Add the egg mixture around the pan until it is even.
5. Reduce the heat and let the omelet cook through.
6. Flip the omelet with a spatula to the other side to cook properly.
7. Roll up or fold the omelet in half to serve.

Nutrition:

- Calories: 104
- Sodium: 34 mg
- Dietary Fiber: 1.4 g
- Total Fat: 4.3 g
- Total Carbs: 14.3 g
- Protein: 1.5 g

116.   Veggie Omelet

Preparation time: 10 minutes

Cooking time: 10 minutes

Servings: 1

Ingredients:

- 4 eggs
- 2 tablespoon olive oil to cook
- 1 small onion, chopped
- 1 bird's eye chili, diced
- A small handful of kale, chopped
- A small handful of arugulas, chopped

Directions:

1. To complete this recipe, you will need to prepare your ingredients. Then, complete the following:
2. Heat olive oil in a frying pan on medium-high heat
3. Cook the onions with the pepper until fragrant and the onions begin to turn translucent. Then, add in the chopped greens. Wait for them to wilt. Then, remove from the pan into a small bowl.
4. Crack eggs into a separate bowl and beat until mixed and combined. Salt and pepper to taste and then add the eggs to the frying pan, careful to spread them evenly.
5. After a minute of cooking, as the bottom of the egg starts to firm up, add the veggie mixture to the pan and spread them out on one half of the omelet. Then, fold the egg over the veggies. Slide onto a plate, cut in half, and serve.

Each half of the omelet serves 1 person.

Nutrition:

- Calories: 234

- Sodium: 35 mg
- Dietary Fiber: 1.4 g
- Total Fat: 4.3 g,
- Total Carbs: 16.2 g
- Protein: 1.3 g

117.   Bacon Sirtfood Omelet

Preparation time: 10 minutes

Cooking time: 20 minutes

Servings: 2

Ingredients:

- 3.5 ounces of sliced smoked bacon
- 5 medium eggs
- 2 ounces of red endive sliced
- 1 ounce of red onions
- 0.5 ounces of parsley, finely chopped
- 2 teaspoons turmeric
- 2 teaspoons extra virgin olive oil

Directions:

1. Break the eggs into a bowl and whisk, add the onions, endive, parsley, and turmeric.
2. Chop the smoked bacon into cubes, add to the egg mixture and mix properly.
3. Heat the olive oil in a non-stick frying pan until hot but not smoking.
4. Add the egg mixture, using a spatula, move it around the pan to start cooking the egg. Kip the bits of cooked egg moving and swirl the raw egg around the pan until the omelet level is even.
5. Reduce the heat and let the omelet cook properly.
6. Ease the spatula around the edges and roll up or fold the omelet to serve.

Nutrition:

- Calories: 103
- Sodium: 34 mg
- Dietary Fiber: 1.4 g
- Total Fat: 4.5 g
- Total Carbs: 14.3 g
- Protein: 1.7 g

118.   Bacon and Arugula Omelet

Preparation time: 10 minutes

Cooking time: 20 minutes

Servings: 1

Ingredients:

- 4 oz. bacon (usually about two slices)
- 6 medium eggs
- 2 cups of kale or arugula (or both), chopped
- 4 tablespoons chopped parsley
- 2 teaspoons turmeric powder
- 1 teaspoon olive oil to cook

Directions:

1. To complete this recipe, you will need to do the following:
2. Start with frying your bacon over medium or medium-high heat. Wait for the bacon to get crispy, then remove from a pan and place to drain the fat.
3. Clean the pan with a paper towel and set aside.
4. Add eggs to a bowl and whisk thoroughly. Then, add your chopped greens, your parsley, and your turmeric. Chop up the bacon and mix them into the mixture as well.
5. Add oil to pan and heat until hot and shimmery, but not smoky.
6. Add the eggs to the pan and swirl it around with the spatula. Continually mix the cooked egg until the raw egg is flat and even. Reduce heat to medium-low and wait for the omelet to finish.
7. Fold in half, remove from pan, cut in half, and serve.

Nutrition:

- Calories: 105
- Sodium: 34 mg

- Dietary Fiber: 1.7 g
- Total Fat: 4.7 g
- Total Carbs: 16.8 g
- Protein: 2.3 g

Chapter 9:   Desserts Recipes

119.   Chocolate Granola

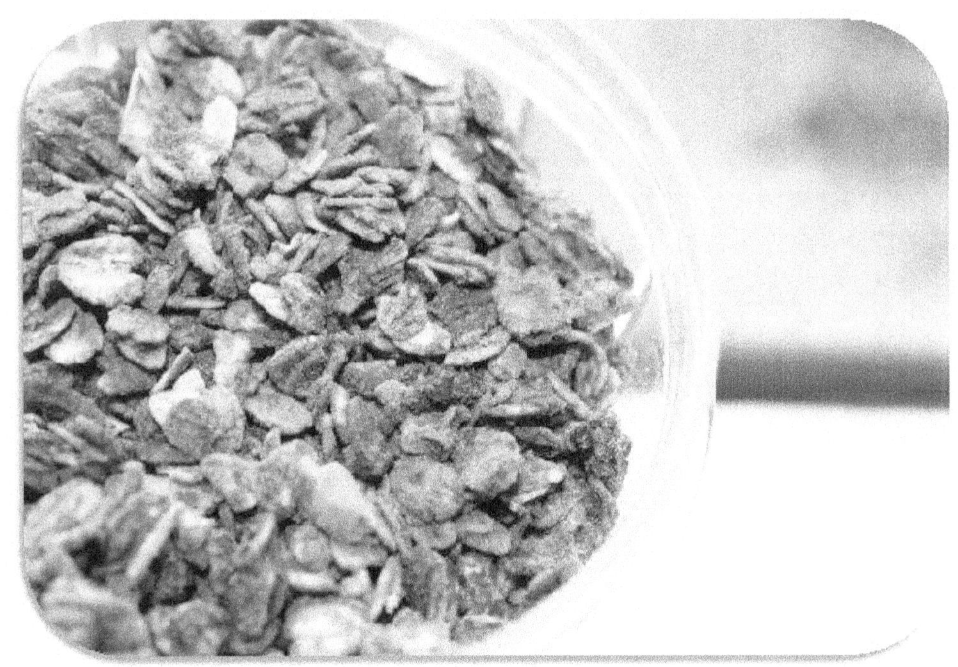

Preparation time: 10 minutes

Cooking time: 38 minutes

Total time: 48 minutes

Servings: 8

Ingredients:

- ¼ cup cacao powder
- ¼ cup maple syrup
- 2 tablespoons coconut oil, melted

- ½ teaspoon vanilla extract
- 1/8 teaspoon salt
- 2 cups gluten-free rolled oats
- ¼ cup unsweetened coconut flakes
- 2 tablespoons chia seeds
- 2 tablespoons unsweetened dark chocolate, chopped finely

Directions:

1. Preheat your oven to 300ºF and line a medium baking sheet with parchment paper.
2. In a medium pan, add the cacao powder, maple syrup, coconut oil, vanilla extract, and salt, and mix well.
3. Now, place the pan over medium heat and cook for about 2–3 minutes, or until thick and syrupy, stirring continuously.
4. Remove from the heat and set aside.
5. In a large bowl, add the oats, coconut, and chia seeds, and mix well.
6. Add the syrup mixture and mix until well combined.
7. Transfer the granola mixture onto a prepared baking sheet and spread in an even layer.
8. Bake for about 35 minutes.
9. Remove from the oven and set aside for about 1 hour.
10. Add the chocolate pieces and stir to combine.
11. Serve immediately.

Nutrition:

- Calories 193
- Sodium: 24 mg
- Dietary Fiber: 1.7 g
- Total Fat: 3.1 g
- Total Carbs: 16.7 g
- Protein: 1.5 g

120.   Homemade Marshmallow Fluff

Preparation time: 10 minutes

Cooking time: 20 minutes

Servings: 2

Ingredients:

- 3/4 cup sugar
- 1/2 cup light corn syrup
- 1/4 cup water
- ⅛ teaspoon salt
- 3 little egg whites
- 1/4 teaspoon cream of tartar
- 1 teaspoon 1/2 tsp vanilla extract

Directions:

1. In a little pan, mix together sugar, corn syrup, salt and water. Attach a candy thermometer into the side of this pan, but make sure it will not touch the underside of the pan.
2. From the bowl of a stand mixer, combine egg whites and cream of tartar. Begin to whip on medium speed with the whisk attachment.
3. Meanwhile, turn a burner on top and place the pan with the sugar mix onto heat. Put the mix into a boil and heat to 240 degrees, stirring periodically.
4. The aim is to have the egg whites whipped to soft peaks and also the sugar heated to 240 degrees at near the same moment. Simply stop stirring the egg whites once they hit soft peaks.
5. Once the sugar has already reached 240 amounts, turn heat low, allowing it to reduce. Insert a little quantity of the popular sugar mix and let it mix. Insert still another little sum of the sugar mix. Add mix slowly and that means you never scramble the egg whites.
6. After all of the sugar was added into the egg whites, then decrease the speed of the mixer and also keep mixing concoction for around 7- 9

minutes until the fluff remains glossy and stiff. At roughly the 5-minute mark, then add the vanilla extract.

7. Use fluff immediately or store in an airtight container in the fridge for around two weeks.

Nutrition:

- Calories: 159
- Sodium: 32 mg
- Dietary Fiber: 1.5 g
- Total Fat: 3.1 g
- Total Carbs: 15.3 g
- Protein: 1.4 g

121. Ultimate Chocolate Chip Cookie N' Oreo Fudge Brownie Bar

Preparation time: 10 minutes

Cooking time: 50 minutes

Servings: 2

Ingredients:

- 1 cup (2 sticks) butter, softened
- 1 cup granulated sugar
- 3/4 cup light brown sugar
- 2 large egg
- 1 tablespoon pure vanilla extract
- 2 ½ cups all-purpose flour
- 1 teaspoon baking soda
- 1 teaspoon lemon
- 2 cups (12 oz) milk chocolate chips
- 1 package double stuffed Oreo
- 1 family-size (9×1 3) brownie mixture
- 1/4 cup hot fudge topping

Directions:

1. Preheat oven to 350 degrees F.
2. Cream the butter and sugars in a large bowl, using an electric mixer at medium speed for 35 minutes.
3. Add the vanilla and eggs and mix well to thoroughly combine. In another bowl, whisk together the flour, baking soda and salt, and slowly incorporate in the mixer everything is combined.
4. Stir in chocolate chips.
5. Spread the cookie dough at the bottom of a 9×1-3 baking dish that is wrapped with wax paper and then coated with cooking spray.
6. Shirt with a coating of Oreos. Mix together brownie mix, adding an optional 1/4 cup of hot fudge directly into the mixture.

7. Stir the brownie batter within the cookie-dough and Oreos.

8. Cover with foil and bake at 350 degrees F for 30 minutes.

9. Remove foil and continue baking for another 15 25 minutes.

10. Let cool before cutting on brownies. They may be gooey at the while warm but will also set up perfectly once chilled.

Nutrition:

- Calories: 145,
- Sodium: 33 mg,
- Dietary Fiber: 1.4 g,
- Total Fat: 4.1 g,
- Total Carbs: 16.7 g,
- Protein: 1.3 g.

122. Crunchy Chocolate Chip Coconut Macadamia Nut Cookies

Preparation time: 20 minutes

Cooking time: 0 minute

Servings: 2

Ingredients:

- 1 cup yogurt
- 1 cup yogurt
- 1/2 teaspoon baking soda
- 1/2 teaspoon salt
- 1 tablespoon of butter, softened
- 1 cup firmly packed brown sugar
- 1/2 cup sugar
- 1 large egg
- 1/2 cup semi-sweet chocolate chips
- 1/2 cup sweetened flaked coconut
- 1/2 cup coarsely chopped dry-roasted macadamia nuts
- 1/2 cup raisins

Directions:

1. Preheat the oven to 325ºf.
2. In a little bowl, whisk together the flour, oats and baking soda and salt, then place aside.
3. In your mixer bowl, mix together the butter/sugar/egg mix.
4. Mix in the flour/oats mix until just combined and stir in the chocolate chips, raisins, nuts, and coconut.
5. Place outsized bits on a parchment-lined cookie sheet.
6. Bake for 1-3 minutes before biscuits are only barely golden brown.
7. Remove from the oven and then leave the cookie sheets to cool at least 10 minutes.

Nutrition:

- Calories: 167
- Sodium: 31 mg
- Dietary Fiber: 1.4 g
- Total Fat: 4.1 g
- Total Carbs: 16.5 g
- Protein: 1.3 g

123.   Walnut & Date Loaf

Preparation Time: 10 minutes

Cooking Time: 15 minutes

Servings: 12

Ingredients:

- 9 ounces of self-rising flour
- 4 ounces of Medrol dates, chopped
- 2 ounces of walnuts, chopped
- 8fl oz. milk
- 3 eggs
- 1 medium banana, mashed
- 1 teaspoon baking soda

Directions:

1. Sieve the baking soda and flour into a bowl.
2. Add in the banana, eggs, milk and dates and combine all the ingredients thoroughly.
3. Transfer the mixture to a lined loaf tin and smooth it out.
4. Scatter the walnuts on top.
5. Bake the loaf in the oven at 180C/360F for 45 minutes.
6. Serve!

Nutrition:

- Calories: 204
- Sodium: 33 mg
- Dietary Fiber: 1.7 g
- Total Fat: 3.1 g
- Total Carbs: 16.5 g
- Protein: 1.4 g

124.   Peach and Blueberry Pie

Preparation time: 1 hour

Cooking time: 0 minute

Servings: 2

Ingredients:

- 1 box of noodle dough

Filling:

- 5 peaches, peeled and chopped (I used roasted peaches)
- 3 cups strawberries
- 3/4 cup sugar
- 1/4 cup bread
- Juice of 1/2 lemon
- 1 egg yolk, beaten

Directions:

1. Preheat oven to 400 degrees.
2. Place dough to a 9-inch pie plate
3. In a big bowl, combine tomatoes, sugar, bread, and lemon juice, then toss to combine. Pour into the pie plate, mounding at the center.
4. Simply take some of the bread and then cut into bits, then put a pie shirt and put the dough in addition to pressing on the edges.
5. Brush crust with egg wash then sprinkles with sugar.
6. Set onto a parchment paper-lined baking sheet.
7. Bake at 400 for about 20 minutes, until crust is browned at borders.
8. Turn oven down to 350, bake for another 40 minutes.
9. Remove and let sit at least 30minutes.
10.   Have with vanilla ice-cream.

Nutrition:

- Calories: 167
- Sodium: 31 mg
- Dietary Fiber: 1.4 g
- Total Fat: 4.1 g
- Total Carbs: 16.6 g
- Protein: 1.2 g

125.   Pear, Cranberry and Chocolate Crisp

Preparation time: 10 minutes

Cooking time: 20 minutes

Servings: 3

Ingredients:

Crumble topping:

- 1/2 cup flour
- 1/2 cup brown sugar
- 1 tsp cinnamon
- ⅛ teaspoon salt
- 3/4 cup yogurt
- 1/4 cup sliced peppers
- 1/3 cup butter, melted
- 1 teaspoon vanilla

Filling:

- 1 tablespoon brown sugar
- 3 teaspoons, cut into balls
- 1/4 cup dried cranberries
- 1 teaspoon lemon juice
- Two handfuls of milk chocolate chips

Directions:

1. Preheat oven to 375.
2. Spray a casserole dish with a butter spray.
3. Put all of the topping ingredients - flour, sugar, cinnamon, salt, nuts, legumes and dried
4. Butter a bowl and then mix. Set aside.
5. In a large bowl, combine the sugar, lemon juice, pears, and cranberries.
6. Once the fully blended move to the prepared baking dish.

7. Spread the topping evenly over the fruit.

8. Bake for about half an hour.

9. Disperse chocolate chips out at the top.

10. Cook for another 10 minutes.

11. Have with ice cream.

Nutrition:

- Calories: 324
- Sodium: 33 mg
- Dietary Fiber: 1.4 g
- Total Fat: 4.1 g
- Total Carbs: 15.3 g
- Protein: 1.3 g

126. Apricot Oatmeal Cookies

Preparation time: 10 minutes

Cooking time: 20 minutes

Servings: 3

Ingredients:

- 1/2 cup (1 stick) butter, softened
- 2/3 cup light brown sugar packed
- 1 egg
- 3/4 cup all-purpose flour
- 1/2 teaspoon baking soda
- 1/2 teaspoon vanilla extract
- 1/2 teaspoon cinnamon
- 1/4 teaspoon salt
- 1 teaspoon 1/2 cups chopped oats
- 3/4 cup yolks
- 1/4 cup sliced apricots
- 1/3 cup slivered almonds

Directions:

1. Preheat oven to 350°.
2. In a big bowl, combine with the butter, sugar, and egg until smooth.
3. In another bowl, whisk the flour, baking soda, cinnamon, and salt together.
4. Stir the dry ingredients to the butter-sugar bowl.
5. Now stir in the oats, raisins, apricots, and almonds.
6. I heard on the web that in this time, it's much better to cool with the dough (therefore, your biscuits are thicker)
7. Afterward, I scooped my biscuits into some parchment-lined (easier removal and wash up) cookie sheet - around two inches apart.
8. Sliced mine for approximately ten minutes - they were fantastic!

Nutrition:

- Calories: 132
- Sodium: 33 mg
- Dietary Fiber: 1.4 g
- Total Fat: 3.1 g
- Total Carbs: 16.4 g
- Protein: 1.3 g

127.   Blueberry Muffins

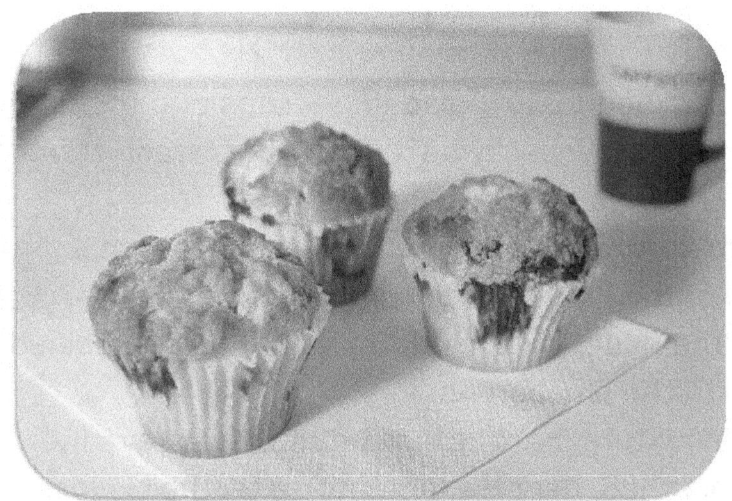

Preparation time: 15 minutes

Cooking time: 20 minutes

Total time: 35 minutes

Servings: 8

Ingredients:

- 1 cup buckwheat flour
- ¼ cup arrowroot starch
- 1½ teaspoons baking powder
- ¼ teaspoon sea salt
- 2 eggs
- ½ cup unsweetened almond milk
- 2–3 tablespoons maple syrup
- 2 tablespoons coconut oil, melted
- 1 cup fresh blueberries

Directions:

1. Preheat your oven to 350ºF and line 8 cups of a muffin tin.
2. In a bowl, place the buckwheat flour, arrowroot starch, baking powder, and salt, and mix well.
3. In a separate bowl, place the eggs, almond milk, maple syrup, and coconut oil, and beat until well combined.
4. Now, place the flour mixture and mix until just combined.
5. Gently, fold in the blueberries.
6. Transfer the mixture into prepared muffin cups evenly.
7. Bake for about 25 minutes or until a toothpick inserted in the center comes out clean.
8. Remove the muffin tin from the oven and place onto a wire rack to cool for about 10 minutes.
9. Carefully invert the muffins onto the wire rack to cool completely before serving.

Nutrition:

- Calories 136
- Sodium: 33 mg
- Dietary Fiber: 2.4 g
- Total Fat: 4.5 g
- Total Carbs: 16.4 g
- Protein: 1.2 g

128. Chocolate Waffles

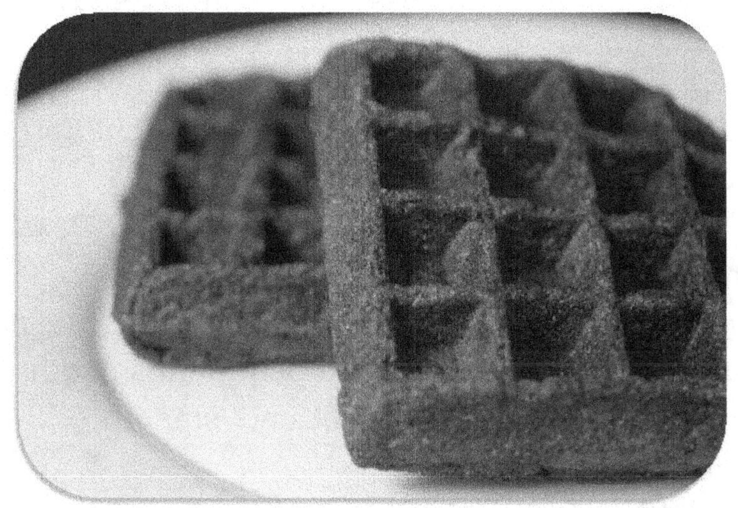

Preparation time: 15 minutes

Cooking time: 24 minutes

Total time: 39 minutes

Servings: 8

Ingredients:

- 2 cups unsweetened almond milk
- 1 tablespoon fresh lemon juice
- 1 cup buckwheat flour
- ½ cup cacao powder
- ¼ cup flaxseed meal
- 1 teaspoon baking soda
- 1 teaspoon baking powder
- ¼ teaspoons kosher salt
- 2 large eggs
- ½ cup coconut oil, melted

- ¼ cup dark brown sugar
- 2 teaspoons vanilla extract
- 2 ounces unsweetened dark chocolate, chopped roughly

Directions:

1. In a bowl, add the almond milk and lemon juice and mix well.
2. Set aside for about 10 minutes.
3. In a bowl, place buckwheat flour, cacao powder, flaxseed meal, baking soda, baking powder, and salt, and mix well.
4. In the bowl of the almond milk mixture, place the eggs, coconut oil, brown sugar, and vanilla extract, and beat until smooth.
5. Now, place the flour mixture and beat until smooth.
6. Gently fold in the chocolate pieces.
7. Preheat the waffle iron and then grease it.
8. Place the desired amount of the mixture into the preheated waffle iron and cook for about 3 minutes, or until golden-brown.
9. Repeat with the remaining mixture.

Nutrition:

- Calories 295
- Sodium: 28 mg
- Dietary Fiber: 1.8 g
- Total Fat: 3.3 g
- Total Carbs: 14.2 g
- Protein: 1.4 g

129.   Snowflakes

Preparation time: 10 minutes

Cooking time: 0 minute

Servings: 2

Ingredients:

- Won ton wrappers
- Oil for frying
- Powdered sugar

Directions:

1. Cut won ton wrappers just like you'd a snowflake
2. Heat oil. When hot, add wonton, fry for approximately 30 seconds, then flips over.
3. Drain on a paper towel and dust with powdered sugar.

Nutrition:

- Calories: 104
- Sodium: 37 mg
- Dietary Fiber: 1.3 g
- Total Fat: 4.6 g
- Total Carbs: 15.6 g
- Protein: 1.5 g

130.   Guilt Totally Free Banana Ice-Cream

Preparation time: 20 minutes

Cooking time: 0 minute

Serves: 3

Ingredients:

- 3 quite ripe banana - peeled and chopped
- A couple of chocolate chips
- 2 tablespoons skim milk

Directions:

1. Throw all ingredients into a food processor and blend until creamy.
2. Eat: freeze and appreciate afterward.

Nutrition:

- Calories: 208
- Sodium: 33 mg
- Dietary Fiber: 1.6 g
- Total Fat: 2.6 g
- Total Carbs: 14.6 g
- Protein: 1.8 g

131.   Pomegranate Guacamole

Preparation time: 10 minutes

Cooking time: 30 minutes

Servings: 1

Ingredients:

- Flesh of 2 ripe avocados
- Seeds from 1 pomegranate
- 1 bird's-eye chili pepper, finely chopped
- ½ red onion, finely chopped
- Juice of 1 lime

Directions:

1. Place the avocado, onion, chill and lime juice into a blender and process until smooth.
2. Stir in the pomegranate seeds. Chill before serving.
3. Serve as a dip for chop vegetables.

Nutrition:

- Calories: 286
- Sodium: 38 mg
- Dietary Fiber: 1.8 g
- Total Fat: 4.3 g
- Total Carbs: 16.5 g
- Protein: 1.7 g

132.   Mascarpone Cheesecake With Almond Crust

Preparation time: 10 minutes

Cooking time: 0 minute

Servings: 2

Ingredients:

- Crust:
- 1/2 cup slivered almonds
- 8 teaspoons or 2/3 cup graham cracker crumbs
- 2 tablespoons sugar
- 1 tablespoon salted butter, melted

Filling:

- 1 (8-ounce) packages cream cheese, room temperature
- 1 (8-ounce) container mascarpone cheese, room temperature
- 3/4 cup sugar
- 1 teaspoon fresh lemon juice (I needed to use imitation lemon-juice)
- 1 teaspoon vanilla extract
- 2 large eggs, room temperature

Directions

1. For the crust: Preheat oven to 350 degrees F. You will need a 9-inch pan (I had a throw off). Finely grind the almonds, cracker crumbs sugar in a food processor (I used my Magical Bullet). Add the butter and process until moist crumbs form.
2. Press the almond mixture on the base of the prepared pan (maybe not on the edges of the pan). Bake the crust until it's set and start to brown, about 1-2 minutes. Cool. Reduce the oven temperature to 325 degrees F.
3. For your filling: with an electric mixer, beat the cream cheese, mascarpone cheese, and sugar in a large bowl until smooth, occasionally scraping down the sides of the jar using a rubber spatula. Beat in the

lemon juice and vanilla. Add the eggs, one at a time, beating until combined after each addition.

4. Pour the cheese mixture on the crust from the pan. Put the pan into a big skillet or Pyrex dish, pour enough hot water to the roasting pan to come halfway up the sides of one's skillet. Bake until the middle of the filling moves slightly when the pan is gently shaken, about 1 hour (the dessert will get hard when it's cold). Transfer the cake to a stand; cool for 1 hour. Refrigerate until the cheesecake is cold, at least eight hours.

5. Topping: squeeze just a small thick cream in the microwave using a chopped Lindt dark chocolate afterward, get a Ziplock baggie and cut out a hole at the corner, then pour the melted chocolate into the baggie and used this to decorate the cake!

Nutrition:

- Calories: 148
- Sodium: 26 mg
- Dietary Fiber: 1.4 g
- Total Fat: 3.1 g
- Total Carbs: 11.2 g
- Protein: 1.6 g

133.   Tofu Guacamole

Preparation time: 10 minutes

Cooking time: 30 minutes

Servings: 1

Ingredients:

- 8oz silken tofu
- 3 avocados
- 2 tablespoons fresh coriander (cilantro) chopped
- 1 bird's-eye chili
- Juice of 1 lime

Directions:

1. Place all of the ingredients into a food processor and blend a soft chunky consistency.
2. Serve with crudités.

Nutrition:

- Calories: 178
- Sodium: 31 mg
- Dietary Fiber: 1.2 g
- Total Fat: 4.1 g
- Total Carbs: 16.6 g
- Protein: 1.4 g

134.   Chocolate Fondue

Preparation Time: 10 minutes

Cooking Time: 15 minutes

Servings: 1

Ingredients:

- 4 ounces of dark chocolate min 85% cocoa
- 11 ounces of strawberries
- 7 ounces of cherries
- 2 apples, peeled, cored and sliced
- 3½ FL oz. double cream, heavy cream

Directions:

1. In a fondue pot or saucepan, place the chocolate and cream then warm it until smooth and creamy.
2. Serve in the fondue pot or transfer it to a serving bowl.
3. Scatter the fruit in a serving dish ready to be dipped into the chocolate.

Nutrition:

- Calories: 220,
- Sodium: 43 mg,
- Dietary Fiber: 5.4 g,
- Total Fat: 2.1 g,
- Total Carbs: 1.3 g,
- Protein: 10.3 g.

135.   Choc Nut Truffles

Preparation Time: 10 minutes

Cooking Time: 15 minutes

Servings: 1

Ingredients:

- 5 ounces of desiccated shredded coconut
- 2 ounces of walnuts, chopped
- 1 ounce of hazelnuts, chopped
- 4 Medjool dates
- 2 tablespoons 100% cocoa powder or cacao nibs
- 1 tablespoon coconut oil

Directions:

1. Place ingredients into a blender and process until smooth and creamy.
2. Using a teaspoon, scoop the mixture into bite-size pieces, then roll it into balls.
3. Place them into small paper cases, cover them and chill for 1 hour before serving.

Nutrition:

- Calories: 220,
- Sodium: 43 mg,
- Dietary Fiber: 5.4 g,
- Total Fat: 2.1 g,
- Total Carbs: 1.3 g,
- Protein: 10.3 g.

136.   No-Bake Strawberry Flapjacks

Preparation Time: 10 minutes

Cooking Time: 0 minutes

Servings: 1

Ingredients

- 3 ounces of porridge oats
- 4 ounces of dates
- 2 ounces of strawberries
- 2 ounces of peanuts, unsalted
- 2 ounces of walnuts
- 1 tablespoon coconut oil
- 2 tablespoons 100% cocoa powder or cacao nibs

Directions:

1. Place the ingredients into a blender and process until they become a soft consistency.
2. Spread the mixture onto a baking sheet or small flat tin.
3. Press the mixture down and smooth it out.
4. Cut it into 8 pieces, ready to serve.
5. You can add an extra sprinkling of cocoa powder to garnish if you wish.

Nutrition:

- Calories: 123
- Sodium: 30 mg
- Dietary Fiber: 1.4 g
- Total Fat: 2.1 g
- Total Carbs: 11.3 g
- Protein: 1.3 g

137.   Dark Chocolate Pretzel Cookies

Preparation time: 10 minutes

Cooking time: 20 minutes

Servings: 2

Ingredients:

- 1 cup yogurt
- 1/2 teaspoon baking soda
- 1/4 teaspoon salt
- 1/4 teaspoon cinnamon
- 4 tablespoons butter (softened/0
- 1/3 cup brown sugar
- 1 egg
- 1/2 teaspoon vanilla
- 1/2 cup dark chocolate chips
- 1/2 cup pretzels, chopped

Directions

1. Preheat oven to 350 degrees.
2. In a medium bowl, whisk together the sugar, butter, vanilla and egg.
3. In another bowl, stir together the flour, baking soda, and salt.
4. Stir the bread mixture in, using all the wet components, along with the chocolate chips and pretzels until just blended.
5. Drop large spoonful of dough on an unlined baking sheet.
6. Bake for 15-17 minutes, or until the bottoms are somewhat all crispy.
7. Allow cooling on a wire rack.

Nutrition:

- Calories: 150
- Sodium: 28 mg
- Dietary Fiber: 1.7 g
- Total Fat: 4.1 g
- Total Carbs: 16.7 g

- Protein: 1.4 g

138.   Matcha With Vanilla

Preparation Time: 5 Minutes,

Cooking time: 0 minutes

Servings: 1

Swap the tasty green matcha and the white tea in this Japanese-style tea or coffee. It's easy to make at home, and it only takes 5 minutes.

Ingredients:

- Seeds from half a vanilla pod
- ½ teaspoon of matcha powder

Directions

1. Heat the kettle, then apply 100ml of water to it. In a tiny cup, pour half the hot water, steam and then transfer the matcha powder and vanilla seeds to the remaining water in the cup.
2. Stir the mixture up to a smooth, slightly smooth and lump-free matcha with a bamboo whisk or mini-electric whisk. In the hot teapot, remove the water and then dump the cooked matcha tea into it. Prefer, with sweet honey or agave.

Nutrition:

- Calories: 210
- Sodium: 34 mg
- Dietary Fiber: 1.4 g
- Total Fat: 4.3 g
- Total Carbs: 15.3 g
- Protein: 1.6 g

139.   Warm Berries & Cream

Preparation Time: 10 minutes

Cooking Time: 15 minutes

Servings: 1

Ingredients:

- 9 ounces of blueberries
- 9 ounces of strawberries
- 3 ounces of. Red currants
- 3ounce of blackberries
- Tablespoons fresh whipped cream
- 1 tablespoon honey

Directions:

1. Mix all ingredients into a bowl.
2. Scoop out a little of the mixture and shape it into a ball.
3. Roll the ball in a little cocoa powder and set aside.
4. Repeat for the remaining mixture. Can be eaten straight away or stored in the fridge.

Nutrition:

- Calories: 193
- Sodium: 32 mg
- Dietary Fiber: 1.4 g
- Total Fat: 4.6 g
- Total Carbs: 16.8 g
- Protein: 1.6 g

140. Home-Made Ice-Cream Drumsticks

Preparation time: 30 minutes

Cooking time: 0 minute

Servings: 2

Ingredients:

- Vanilla ice cream
- Two Lindt hazelnut chunks
- Magical shell - out chocolate
- Sugar levels
- Nuts (I mixed crushed peppers and unsalted peanuts)
- Parchment paper

Directions:

1. Soften ice cream and mixing topping and two sliced of hazelnut balls.
2. Fill underside of Magic shell with sugar and nuts and top with ice-cream.
3. Wrap parchment paper round cone and then fill cone over about 1.5 inches across the cap of the cone (the paper can help to carry its shape).
4. Sprinkle with magical nuts and shells.
5. Freeze for about 20 minutes, before the ice cream is eaten.

Nutrition:

- Calories: 153
- Sodium: 32 mg
- Dietary Fiber: 1.4 g
- Total Fat: 4.1 g
- Total Carbs: 16.3 g
- Protein: 1.6 g

Chapter 10:   Juice and Smoothies Recipes

141.   Matcha Green Juice

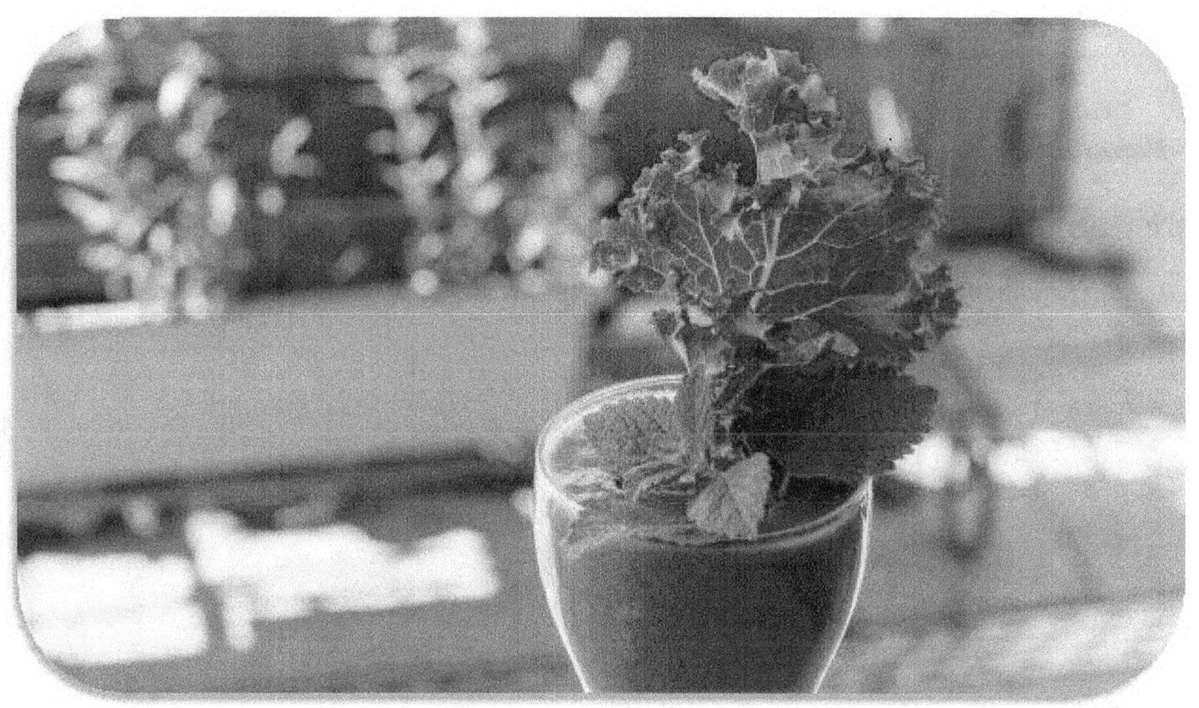

Preparation time: 10 minutes

Cooking time: 0 minutes

Total time: 10 minutes

Servings: 2

Ingredients:

- 5 ounces fresh kale
- 2 ounces fresh arugula
- ¼ cup fresh parsley

- 4 celery stalks
- 1 green apple, cored and chopped
- 1 (1-inch) piece fresh ginger, peeled
- 1 lemon, peeled
- ½ teaspoon matcha green tea

Directions:

1. Add all ingredients into a juicer and extract the juice according to the manufacturer's method.
2. Pour into 2 glasses and serve immediately.

Nutrition:

- Calories: 113
- Sodium: 22 mg
- Dietary Fiber: 1.2 g
- Total Fat: 2.1 g
- Total Carbs: 12.3 g
- Protein: 1.3 g

142. Celery Juice

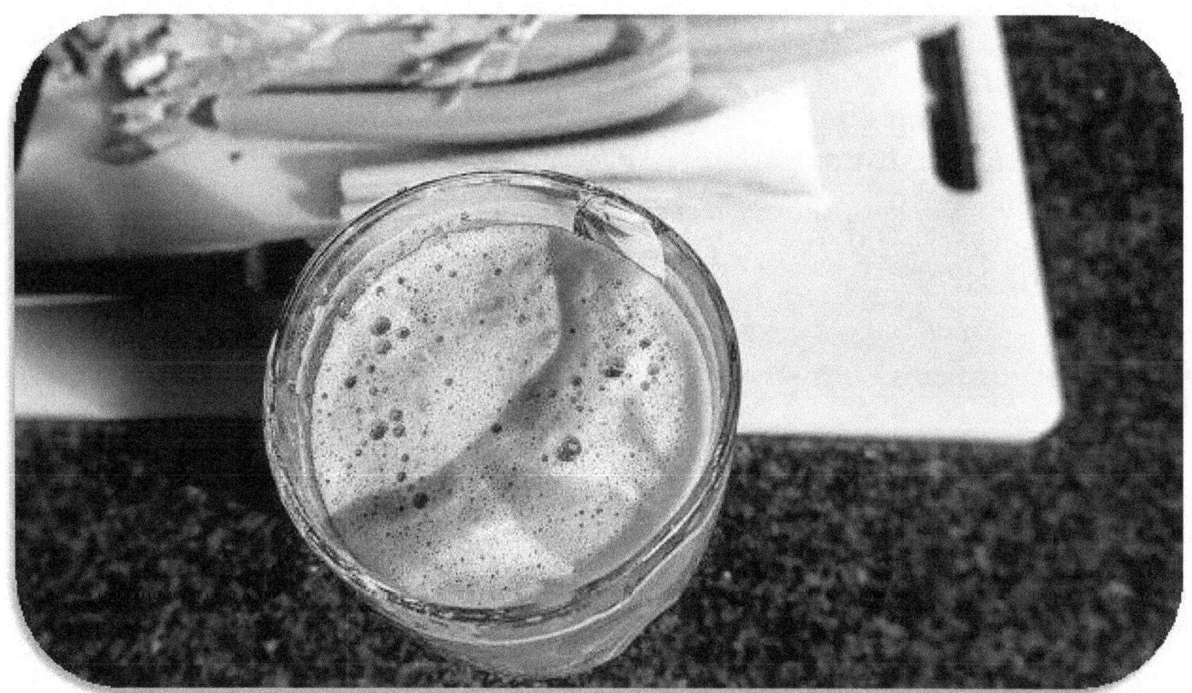

Preparation time: 10 minutes

Cooking time: 0 minutes

Servings: 2

Ingredients:

- 8 celery stalks with leaves
- 2 tablespoons fresh ginger, peeled
- 1 lemon, peeled
- ½ cup filtered water
- Pinch of salt

Instructions:

1. Place all the ingredients in a blender and pulse until well combined.

2. Through a fine mesh strainer, strain the juice and transfer into 2 glasses.
3. Serve immediately.

Nutrition:

- Calories: 32
- Sodium: 21 mg
- Dietary Fiber: 1.4 g
- Total Fat: 1.1 g
- Total Carbs: 1.3 g
- Protein: 1.2 g

143.　Kale & Orange Juice

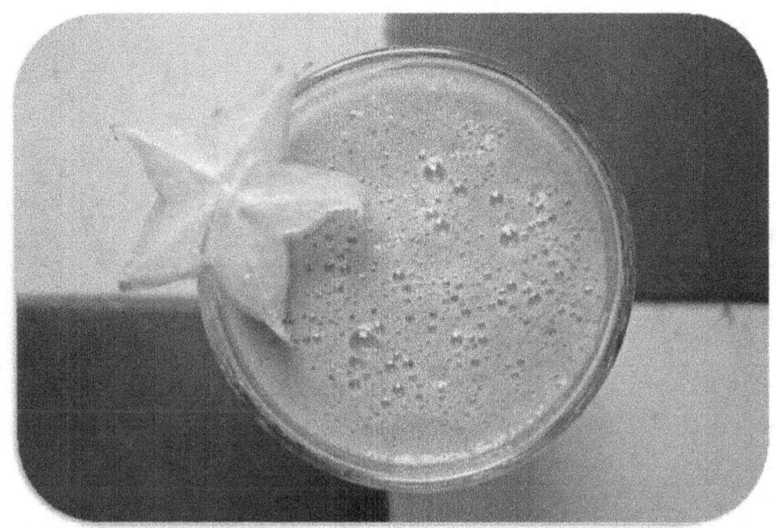

Preparation time: 10 minutes

Cooking time: 0 minutes

Servings: 2

Ingredients:

- 5 large oranges, peeled
- 2 bunches fresh kale

Directions:

1. Add all ingredients into a juicer and extract the juice according to the manufacturer's method.
2. Pour into 2 glasses and serve immediately.

Nutrition:

- Calories: 315
- Sodium: 34 mg
- Dietary Fiber: 1.3 g
- Total Fat: 4.1 g
- Total Carbs: 14.3 g
- Protein: 1.2 g

144.   Apple & Cucumber Juice

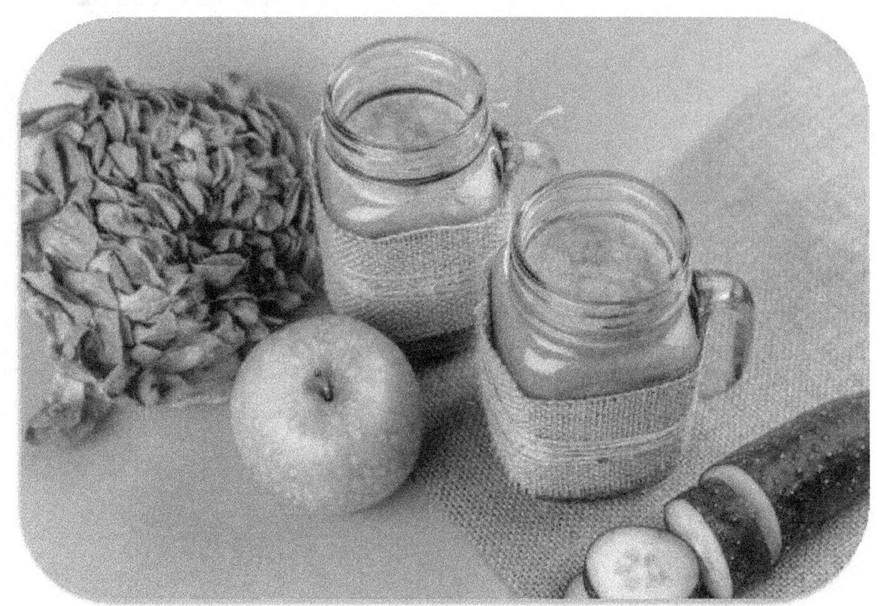

Preparation time: 10 minutes

Cooking time: 0 minutes

Servings: 2

Ingredients:

- 3 large apples, cored and sliced
- 2 large cucumbers, sliced
- 4 celery stalks
- 1 (1-inch) piece fresh ginger, peeled
- 1 lemon, peeled

Directions:

1. Add all ingredients into a juicer and extract the juice according to the manufacturer's method.
2. Pour into 2 glasses and serve immediately.

Nutrition:

- Calories: 230
- Sodium: 31 mg
- Dietary Fiber: 1.3 g
- Total Fat: 2.1 g
- Total Carbs: 1.3 g
- Protein: 1.2 g

145. Lemony Green Juice

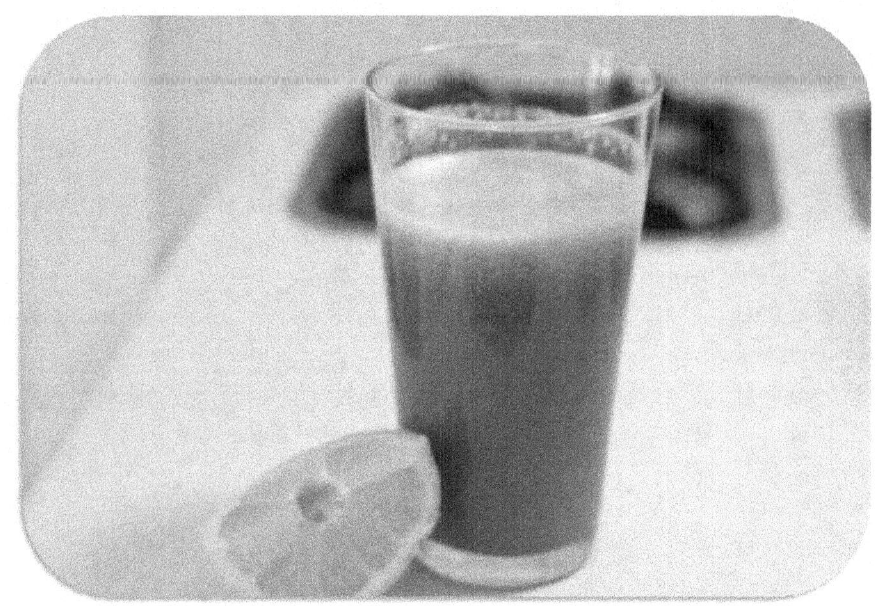

Preparation time: 10 minutes

Cooking time: 0 minutes

Servings: 2

Ingredients:

- 2 large green apples, cored and sliced
- 4 cups fresh kale leaves
- 4 tablespoons fresh parsley leaves
- 1 tablespoon fresh ginger, peeled
- 1 lemon, peeled
- ½ cup filtered water
- Pinch of salt

Directions:

1. Place all the ingredients in a blender and pulse until well combined.
2. Through a fine mesh strainer, strain the juice and transfer into 2 glasses.
3. Serve immediately.

Nutrition:

- Calories: 196
- Sodium: 21 mg
- Dietary Fiber: 1.4 g
- Total Fat: 1.1 g
- Total Carbs: 1.6 g
- Protein: 1.5 g

146.   Orange & Celery Crush

Preparation Time: 10 minutes

Cooking Time: 15 minutes

Servings: 1

Ingredients:

- 1 carrot, peeled
- Stalks of celery
- 1 orange, peeled
- ½ teaspoon matcha powder
- Juice of 1 lime

Directions:

1. Place ingredients into a blender with enough water to cover them and blitz until smooth.

Nutrition:

- Calories: 150
- Sodium: 31 mg
- Dietary Fiber: 1.2 g
- Total Fat: 2.1 g
- Total Carbs: 11.2 g
- Protein: 1.4 g

147.   Creamy Strawberry & Cherry Smoothie

Preparation Time: 10 minutes

Cooking Time: 15 minutes

Servings: 1

Ingredients:

- 3½ ounces of strawberries
- 3.5 ounces of frozen pitted cherries
- 1 tablespoon plain full-fat yogurt
- 6.5 ounces of unsweetened soya milk

Directions:

1. Place the ingredients into a blender, then process until smooth.
2. Serve and enjoy.

Nutrition:

- Calories: 203
- Sodium: 23 mg
- Dietary Fiber: 1.4 g
- Total Fat: 3.1 g
- Total Carbs: 12.3 g
- Protein: 1.7 g

148. Tropical Chocolate Delight

Preparation Time: 10 minutes

Cooking Time: 15 minutes

Servings: 1

Ingredients:

- 1 mango, peeled & de-stoned
- Ounce fresh pineapple, chopped
- 2 ounces of kale
- 1 ounce of rocket
- 1 tablespoon 100% cocoa powder or cacao nibs
- 1 ounce of coconut milk

Direction

1. Place ingredients into a blender and blitz until smooth.
2. You can add a little water if it seems too thick.

Nutrition:

- Calories: 192
- Sodium: 26 mg
- Dietary Fiber: 1.3 g
- Total Fat: 4.1 g
- Total Carbs: 16.6 g
- Protein: 1.6 g

149.   Grapefruit & Celery Blast

Preparation Time: 10 minutes

Cooking Time: 15 minutes

Servings: 1

Ingredients:

- 1 grapefruit, peeled
- stalks of celery
- 2-ounces kale
- ½ teaspoon matcha powder

Directions:

1. Place ingredients into a blender with water to cover them and blitz until smooth.

Nutrition:

- Calories: 129
- Sodium: 24 mg
- Dietary Fiber: 1.4 g
- Total Fat: 2.1 g
- Total Carbs: 12.1 g
- Protein: 1.2 g

150.   Matcha Green Tea Smoothie

Preparation Time: 3 minutes

Cooking time: 0 minute

Serves: 2

Ingredients:

- 2 ripe bananas 2
- 2 teaspoons matcha green tea powder
- 2 teaspoons honey
- 1/2 teaspoon vanilla bean paste (not extract) or a small scrape of the seeds from a vanilla pod
- 250 ml of milk
- Six ice cubes

Directions:

1. Blend all the ingredients in a blender and serve in two glasses.

Nutrition:

- Calories: 183
- Sodium: 26 mg
- Dietary Fiber: 1.4 g
- Total Fat: 2.1 g
- Total Carbs: 12.1 g
- Protein: 1.2 g

151.   Green Tea Smoothie

Preparation time: 10 minutes

Cooking time: 0 minutes

Servings: 1

Ingredients:

- 1 ripe large banana
- Milk
- ¼ teaspoon vanilla bean paste
- 3 ice cubes
- 1 teaspoon honey

Direction

1. Blend all the ingredients together in a blender and serve in a glass.

Nutrition:

- Calories: 185
- Sodium: 21 mg
- Dietary Fiber: 1.3 g
- Total Fat: 2.1 g
- Total Carbs: 10.3 g
- Protein: 1.2 g

152.   Chocolate Balls

Preparation Time: 10 minutes

Cooking Time: 15 minutes

Servings: 1

Ingredients:

- 2 ounces of peanut butter or almond butter
- 1 ounce of cocoa powder
- 1 ounce of desiccated shredded coconut
- 1 tablespoon honey
- 1 tablespoon cocoa powder for coating

Directions:

1. Mix all ingredients into a bowl. Scoop out a little of the mixture and shape it into a ball.
2. Roll the ball in a little cocoa powder and set aside.
3. Repeat for the remaining mixture. Can be eaten straight away or stored in the fridge.

Nutrition:

- Calories: 295
- Sodium: 24 mg
- Dietary Fiber: 1.4 g
- Total Fat: 4.1 g
- Total Carbs: 16.3 g
- Protein: 1.3 g

153. Strawberry & Citrus Blend

Preparation Time: 10 minutes

Cooking Time: 15 minutes

Servings: 1

Ingredients:

- 3 ounces of strawberries
- 1 apple, cored
- 1 orange, peeled
- ½ avocado, peeled and de-stoned
- ½ teaspoon matcha powder
- Juice of 1 lime

Directions:

1. Place ingredients into a blender with enough water to cover them and process until smooth.

Nutrition:

- Calories: 124
- Sodium: 31 mg
- Dietary Fiber: 1.4 g
- Total Fat: 2.1 g
- Total Carbs: 12.2 g
- Protein: 1.2 g

154.   Turmeric Tea

Preparation time: 10 minutes

Servings: 1

Ingredients:

- 1 ½ heaped teaspoon turmeric powder
- ½ tablespoon fresh ginger, grated
- 1 small lemon
- Orange zest
- 1 teaspoon honey.

Directions

1. Boil 200ml of water in the kettle
2. Put the turmeric, ginger, and orange zest in a teapot or jug. Pour over the boiling water and allow to stand for 5 minutes.
3. Strain through a sieve or tea strainer into a cup, add lemon juice or a slice of lemon and sweeten with honey.

Nutrition:

- Calories: 83
- Sodium: 21 mg
- Dietary Fiber: 1.4 g
- Total Fat: 1.1 g
- Total Carbs: 1.3 g
- Protein: 1.2 g

155.   Strawberry and Blackcurrant Jelly

Preparation time: 10 minutes

Cooking time: 0 minute

Servings: 2

Ingredients:

- Strawberries, hulled and chopped
- Blackcurrants washed and stalks removed
- Water
- 3 tablespoons granulated sugar.
- 4 gelatin leaves

Directions:

1. Arrange the strawberries in 4 serving dishes.
2. Put the gelatin leaves in a bowl of cold water to soften.
3. Place the blackcurrants in a small pan with sugar and 200ml of water and boil. Simmer vigorously for 5 minutes and then remove from heat. Leave to stand for 2 minutes
4. Squeeze out excess water from the gelatin leaves and add them to the blackcurrant mixture. Stir until fully dissolved, then stir in the rest of the water.
5. Pour the liquid into the prepared dishes and refrigerate till it set. The jelly should be ready in about 3 to 4 hours or you can leave it overnight.

Nutrition:

- Calories: 232
- Sodium: 24 mg
- Dietary Fiber: 1.4 g
- Total Fat: 2.1 g
- Total Carbs: 10.3 g
- Protein: 1.2 g

156.   Green Juice Salad

Preparation time: 10 minutes

Cooking time: 0 minute

Servings: 1

Ingredients:

- 2 handfuls of chopped kale
- 1 handful of chopped arugulas
- 1 tablespoon chopped parsley
- 2 stalks of celery, sliced into bite-sized pieces
- ½ green apple, chopped into bite-sized pieces
- 6 walnuts, crushed
- 1 tablespoon olive oil
- ½ lemon, juiced
- 1 teaspoon grated ginger
- A pinch of salt and pepper

Directions:

1. To complete this recipe, you will need to do the following:
2. Mix the juice of the lemon, ginger, seasonings, and olive oil into a small jar or small Tupperware container. Set aside until you are ready to eat.
3. In a large bowl or large Tupperware container, add your kale, arugula, parsley, celery, apple, and walnut. Mix it up until well combined and set aside until you are ready to eat.
4. When you are ready to eat it, shake up your dressing, then add it to the bowl and mix thoroughly.

Nutrition:

- Calories: 385
- Sodium: 32 mg
- Dietary Fiber: 1.2 g
- Total Fat: 4.1 g
- Total Carbs: 12.3 g

- Protein: 1.3 g

157. Sirtfood Smoothie

Preparation time: 10 minutes

Cooking time: 0 minutes

Servings: 2

Ingredients:

- 3 ounces of plain Greek yogurt (or vegan alternative, such as soy or coconut yogurt)
- 6 walnut halves
- 10 medium strawberries, hulled
- A handful of kale stalks removed
- 1 ounce of dark chocolate (85 percent cocoa solids)
- 1 Medjool date, pitted
- 1/2 teaspoon ground turmeric
- 1 small size chili
- 7/8 cup (200ml) unsweetened almond milk.
- 1 teaspoon honey

Directions:

1. Blend all the ingredients in a blender until smooth and serve in a glass.

Nutrition:

- Calories: 162,
- Sodium: 28 mg,
- Dietary Fiber: 1.4 g,
- Total Fat: 3.1 g,
- Total Carbs: 11.3 g,
- Protein: 1.2 g.

158. Centrifuged Green Juice

Preparation time: 10 minutes

Cooking time: 0 minutes

Servings: 2

Ingredients:

- 1.3 ounce of kale
- 1.5 ounce of rocket salad
- 0.7 ounce of parsley
- 5 ounces of green celery with the leaves
- 1/2 green apple
- 1/2 lemon juice
- 1/2 teaspoon of matcha tea

Directions:

1. Centrifuge the kale, rocket salad and parsley; add grated celery and apple; enrich with half a squeezed lemon and half a teaspoon of matcha tea.
2. Drink immediately so as not to lose the beneficial effects of vegetables and not keep it in the fridge. It should always be prepared when consuming it.

Nutrition:

- Calories: 150
- Sodium: 32 mg
- Dietary Fiber: 1.4 g
- Total Fat: 2.1 g
- Total Carbs: 7.3 g
- Protein: 1.2 g

159. Iced Cranberry Green Juice

Preparation time: 10 minutes

Cooking time: 30 minutes

Servings: 1

Ingredients:

- 5fl Oz light cranberry juice
- 3½fl Oz green tea, cooled
- Squeeze of lemon juice
- A handful of crushed ice (optional)
- Sprig of mint

Directions:

1. Pour the green tea and cranberry into a glass and add a squeeze of lemon juice.
2. Top it off with some ice and garnish with a mint leaf.

Nutrition:

- Calories: 14
- Sodium: 23 mg
- Dietary Fiber: 1.4 g
- Total Fat: 2.1 g
- Total Carbs: 1.3 g
- Protein: 1.2 g

160. Ginger & Turmeric Juice

Preparation time: 10 minutes

Cooking time: 7 minutes

Servings: 1

Ingredients:

- 1-inch chunk fresh ginger root, peeled
- ¼ teaspoon turmeric
- 1 teaspoon of honey (optional)
- Ice

Directions

1. Make incisions in the piece of root ginger, without cutting all the way through.
2. Place the ginger and turmeric in a cup and pour in boiling water. Allow it to steep for 7 minutes.
3. Add a teaspoon of honey if you wish. Let it cook and then add ice and enjoy.

Nutrition:

- Calories: 33
- Sodium: 22 mg
- Dietary Fiber: 1.6 g
- Total Fat: 1.1g
- Total Carbs: 1.3 g
- Protein: 1.2 g

Chapter 11:   Snacks Recipes

161.   Homemade Hummus & Celery

Preparation time: 10 minutes

Cooking time: 40 minutes

Servings: 1

Ingredients:

- 8 sticks of celery, cut into batons
- 6oz tinned chickpeas (garbanzo beans), drained
- 2 cloves of garlic, crushed
- 1 tablespoon fresh parsley, chopped
- 1 tablespoon tahini (sesame seed paste)
- Juice of 1 lemon
- 1 tablespoon olive oil

Directions:

1. Place the chickpeas (garbanzo beans) into a blender along with the garlic, tahini pastes and lemon juice. Process until it's smooth and creamy.
2. Transfer the mixture to a serving bowl.
3. Make a small well in the center of the dip and pour in the olive oil.
4. Sprinkle with parsley. Serve the celery sticks on a plate alongside the hummus.

Nutrition:

- Calories: 412
- Sodium: 33 mg
- Dietary Fiber: 1.8 g
- Total Fat: 5.1 g
- Total Carbs: 16.8 g
- Protein: 1.3 g

162.   Rosemary & Garlic Kale Chips

Preparation time: 10 minutes

Cooking time: 30 minutes

Servings: 1

Ingredients:

- 9oz kale chips, chopped into 2inch
- 2 sprigs of rosemary
- 2 cloves of garlic
- 2 tablespoons olive oil
- Sea salt
- Freshly ground black pepper

Directions:

1. Gently warm the olive oil, rosemary and garlic over a low heat for 10 minutes. Remove it from the heat and set aside to cool.
2. Take the rosemary and garlic out of the oil and discard them.
3. Toss the kale leaves in the oil, making sure they are well coated.
4. Season with salt and pepper.
5. Spread the kale leaves onto 2 baking sheets and bake them in the oven at 170C/325F for 15 minutes, until crispy.

Nutrition:

- Calories: 249
- Sodium: 36 mg
- Dietary Fiber: 1.7 g
- Total Fat: 4.3 g
- Total Carbs: 15.3 g
- Protein: 1.4 g

163.   Strawberry Frozen Yogurt

Preparation Time: 10 minutes

Cooking Time: 15 minutes

Servings: 4

Ingredients:

- 15 ounces of plain yogurt
- 6 ounces of strawberries
- Juice of 1 orange
- 1 tablespoon honey

Directions:

1. Place the strawberries and orange juice into a food processor or blender and blitz until smooth.
2. Press the mixture through a sieve into a large bowl to remove seeds.
3. Stir in the honey and yogurt. Transfer the mixture to an ice-cream maker and follow the manufacturer's instructions.
4. Alternatively, pour the mixture into a container and place in the fridge for 1 hour. Use a fork to whisk it and break up the ice crystals and freeze for 2 hours.

Nutrition:

- Calories: 238
- Sodium: 33 mg
- Dietary Fiber: 1.4 g
- Total Fat: 1.8 g
- Total Carbs: 12.3 g
- Protein: 1.3 g

164.   Berry Soy Yogurt Parfait

Preparation time: 2-4 minutes

Cooking time: 0 minute

Servings: 1

Ingredients:

- 1cartonvanillacultured soy yogurt
- 1/4 cup granola (gluten-free)
- 1 cup berries (you can take strawberries, blueberries, raspberries, blackberries)

Directions:

1. Put half of the yogurt in a glass jar or serving dish.
2. On the top put half of the berries.
3. Then sprinkle with half of granola
4. Repeat layers.

Nutrition:

- Calories: 244
- Sodium: 33 mg
- Dietary Fiber: 1.4 g
- Total Fat: 3.1 g
- Total Carbs: 11.3 g
- Protein: 1.4 g

165.   Walnut & Spiced Apple Tonic

Preparation Time: 10 minutes

Cooking Time: 15 minutes

Servings: 1

Ingredients:

- 6 walnuts halves
- 1 apple, cored
- 1 banana
- ½ teaspoon matcha powder
- ½ teaspoon cinnamon
- Pinch of ground nutmeg

Directions:

1. Place ingredients into a blender and add sufficient water to cover them. Blitz until smooth and creamy.

Nutrition:

- Calories: 124
- Sodium: 22 mg
- Dietary Fiber: 1.4 g
- Total Fat: 2.1 g
- Total Carbs: 12.3 g
- Protein: 1.2 g

166. Basil & Walnut Pesto

Preparation time: 10 minutes

Cooking time: 30 minutes

Servings: 1

Ingredients:

- 2oz fresh basil
- 2oz walnuts
- 1oz pine nuts
- 3 cloves of garlic, crushed
- 2 tablespoons Parmesan, grated
- 4 tablespoons olive oil

Direction

1. Place the pesto ingredients into a food processor and process until it becomes a smooth paste.
2. Serve with meat, fish, salad and pasta dishes.

Nutrition

- Calories: 136
- Sodium: 23 mg,
- Dietary Fiber: 1.2 g,
- Total Fat: 3.1 g,
- Total Carbs: 14.3 g
- Protein: 1.4 g

167.   Honey Chili Nuts

Preparation time: 10 minutes

Cooking time: 30 minutes

Servings: 1

Ingredients:

- 5oz walnuts
- 5oz pecan nuts
- 2oz softened butter
- 1 tablespoon honey
- ½ bird's-eye chili, very finely chopped and de-seeded

Directions

1. Preheat the oven to 180C/360F.
2. Combine the butter, honey and chili in a bowl, then add the nuts and stir them well.
3. Spread the nuts onto a lined baking sheet and roast them in the oven for 10 minutes, stirring once halfway through.
4. Remove from the oven and allow them to cool before eating.

Nutrition:

- Calories: 295
- Sodium: 28 mg
- Dietary Fiber: 1.6 g
- Total Fat: 4.7 g
- Total Carbs: 14.6 g
- Protein: 1.3 g

168.   Lemon Ricotta Cookies With Lemon Glaze

Preparation time: 20 minutes

Cooking time: 30 minutes

Servings: 2

Ingredients:

- 2 ½ cups all-purpose flour
- 1 teaspoon baking powder
- 1 teaspoon salt
- 1 tablespoon unsalted butter, softened
- 2 cups of sugar
- 2 eggs
- 1 teaspoon (15-ounce) container whole-milk ricotta cheese
- 3 tablespoons lemon juice
- Zest of one lemon

Glaze:

- 1/2 cups powdered sugar
- 3 tablespoons lemon juice
- Zest of one lemon

Directions:

1. Preheat the oven to 375 degrees f.
2. In a medium bowl, combine the flour, baking powder and salt. Set-aside.
3. From the big bowl, blend the butter and the sugar together. With an electric mixer, beat the sugar and butter until light and fluffy, about three minutes. Add the eggs, one at a time, beating until incorporated.
4. Insert the ricotta cheese, lemon juice, and lemon zest. Beat to blend. Stir in the dry ingredients.
5. Line two baking sheets with parchment paper. Spoon the dough (approximately 2 tablespoons of each cookie) on the baking sheets. Bake for 15 minutes, until slightly golden at the borders. Remove from the

oven and allow the cookies to remain on the baking sheet for about 20 minutes.

Glaze:

1. Combine the powdered sugar, lemon juice and lemon zest in a small bowl and then stir until smooth.
2. Spoon approximately 1/2-tsp on each cookie and use of the back of the spoon to lightly disperse.
3. Allow glaze to harden for approximately two hours.
4. Pack the biscuits in a decorative jar.

Nutrition:

- Calories: 156
- Sodium: 28 mg
- Dietary Fiber: 1.4 g
- Total Fat: 5.1 g
- Total Carbs: 16.8
- Protein: 1.2 g

169.   Perfect Little PB Snack Balls

Preparation time: 10 minutes

Cooking time: 20 minutes

Servings: 2

Ingredients:

- 1/2 cup chunky peanut butter
- 3 tablespoons flax seeds
- 3 tablespoons wheat germs
- 1 tablespoon honey or agave
- 1/4 cup powdered sugar

Directions:

1. Blend dry ingredients and adding from the honey and peanut butter.
2. Mix well and roll into chunks and then conclude by rolling into wheat germ.

Nutrition:

- Calories: 124
- Sodium: 28 mg
- Dietary Fiber: 1.7 g
- Total Fat: 2.3 g
- Total Carbs: 11.3 g
- Protein: 1.3 g

170.   Spaghetti With Tomato, Vanilla and Fried Capers

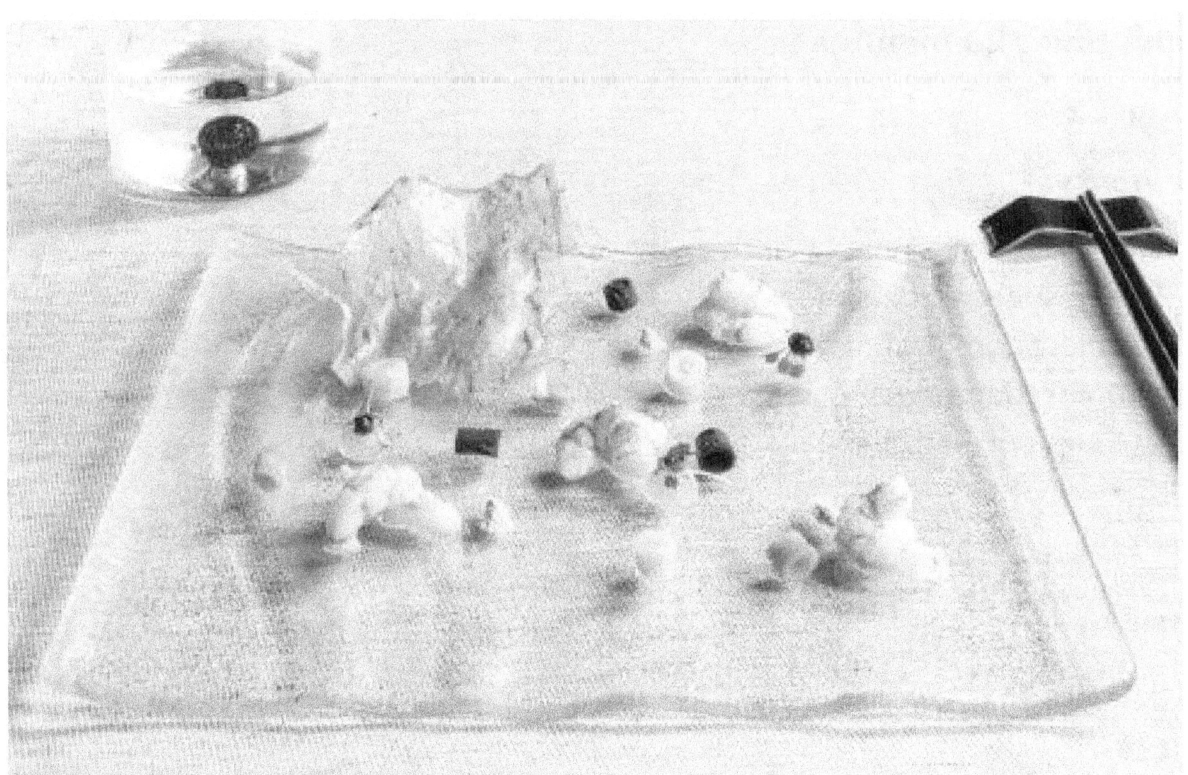

Preparation time: 10 Minutes,

Cooking time: 30 Minutes,

Servings: 4

Ingredients:

- Tomato sauce
- 4 dried tomatoes
- 1 handful of salted capers
- 1 vanilla bean
- Garlic
- Oil
- Salt
- Pepper

- Paprika
- Peanut oil
- Spaghetti

Directions:

1. Desalt the capers by soaking them for 10 minutes. Squeeze well, then pass in a hot pan, lukewarm, to evaporate all the water. Bring the seed oil to temperature: dip the capers, let them explode and take them, taking care to pass them on the absorbent paper without pressing.
2. In the meantime, heat a pan well and rub the peeled garlic on the bottom. Pour two tablespoons of oil and leave to flavor. Add the tomato puree to the warm oil. Open the vanilla pod, remove the seeds and add them to the tomato. Flavor it with pepper and a splash of paprika. Drop the spaghetti.
3. Cut the sun-dried tomatoes into strips. Add to the sauce. Sprinkle with pepper and paprika. Drain the spaghetti, and finish cooking for two minutes in the pan with the sauce. Roll and place on plates, sprinkling with fried capers.

Nutrition:

- Calories: 200
- Sodium: 30 mg
- Dietary Fiber: 1.4 g
- Total Fat: 3.1 g
- Total Carbs: 14.3
- Protein: 1.6 g

171. Marshmallow Popcorn Balls

Preparation time: 10 minutes

Cooking time: 20 minutes

Servings: 2

Ingredients:

- 2 bags of microwave popcorn
- 1 12.6 ounces. Tote M&M's
- 3 cups honey roasted peanuts
- 1 pkg. 16 ounces. Massive marshmallows
- 1 cup butter, cubed

Directions

1. In a bowl, blend the popcorn, peanuts and M&M's.
2. In a big pot, combine marshmallows and butter.
3. Cook using medium-low heat.
4. Insert popcorn mix, blend thoroughly
5. Spray muffin tins with non-stick cooking spray.
6. When cool enough to handle, spray hands together with non-stick cooking spray and then shape into chunks and put into the muffin tin to shape.
7. Add Popsicle stick into each chunk and then let cool.
8. Wrap each serving in vinyl when chilled.

Nutrition:

- Calories: 104
- Sodium: 27 mg
- Dietary Fiber: 1.4 g
- Total Fat: 2.1 g
- Total Carbs: 10.1 g
- Protein: 1.3 g

172.   Baby Spinach Snack

Preparation time: 10 minutes

Cooking time: 10 minutes

Servings: 3

Ingredients:

- 2 cups baby spinach, washed
- A pinch of black pepper
- ½ tablespoon olive oil
- ½ teaspoon garlic powder

Directions:

1. Spread the baby spinach on a lined baking sheet, add oil, black pepper and garlic powder, toss a bit.
2. Introduce in the oven, bake at 350 degrees F for 10 minutes.
3. Divide into bowls and serve as a snack.

Nutrition:

- Calories: 125
- Sodium: 33 mg
- Dietary Fiber: 1.4 g
- Total Fat: 2.1 g
- Total Carbs: 11.2 g
- Protein: 1.7 g

173.   Potato Bites

Preparation time: 10 minutes

Cooking time: 20 minutes

Servings: 3

Ingredients:

- 1 potato, sliced
- 2 bacon slices, already cooked and crumbled
- 1 small avocado, pitted and cubed
- Cooking spray

Directions:

1. Spread potato slices on a lined baking sheet, spray with cooking oil.
2. Introduce in the oven at 350 degrees F, bake for 20 minutes, arrange on a platter, top each slice with avocado and crumbled bacon and serve as a snack.

Enjoy!

Nutrition:

- Calories: 180
- Sodium: 28 mg
- Dietary Fiber: 1.4 g
- Total Fat: 3.1 g
- Total Carbs: 14.3 g
- Protein: 1.8 g

174.   Thyme Mushrooms

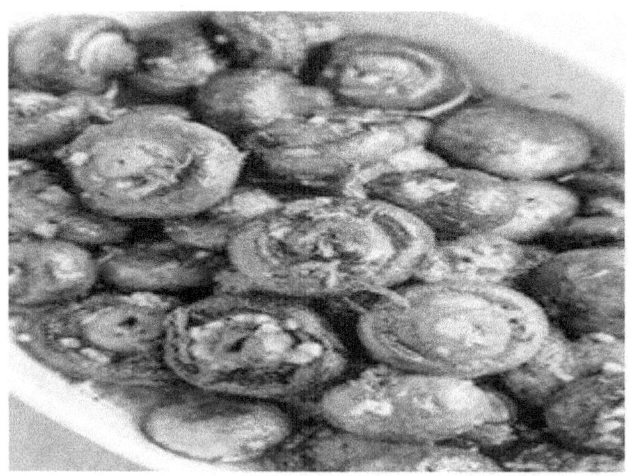

Preparation time: 10 minutes

Cooking time: 45 minutes

Servings: 2

Ingredients:

- 1 tablespoon chopped thyme
- 2 tablespoons olive oil
- 2 tablespoons chopped parsley
- 4 minced garlic cloves
- Black pepper
- 2 lbs. halved white mushrooms

Directions:

1. In a baking pan, combine the mushrooms with the garlic and the other ingredients, toss, introduce in the oven and cook at 400 0F for 30 minutes.
2. Divide between plates and serve.

Nutrition:

- Calories: 251
- Sodium: 37 mg
- Dietary Fiber: 1.3 g
- Total Fat: 3.1 g
- Total Carbs: 15.3 g
- Protein: 1.4 g

175.   Sautéed Mushroom

Preparation time: 10 minutes

Cooking time: 20 minutes

Servings: 2

Ingredients:

- 1/2 Pound mushroom, wiped clean with a wet paper towel
- 2 tablespoons extra-virgin olive oil
- 2 teaspoons fresh lemon juice
- ¼ cup chopped parsley
- 1 small chili, finely chopped.
- ½ teaspoon turmeric

Directions:

1. Cut off mushroom stems. With a small sharp knife, cut grooves on each mushroom that spiral out from the center to edges.
2. Heat the olive oil in the skillet until hot, add mushrooms, fluted side down, veins up. Add lemon juice and turmeric, cook gently for 4 to 5 minutes, then turn over and cook briefly.
3. Sprinkle with parsley and the chili, stir. Serve immediately

Nutrition:

- Calories: 204
- Sodium: 33 mg
- Dietary Fiber: 1.3 g
- Total Fat: 2.3 g
- Total Carbs: 16.2 g
- Protein: 1.3 g

176.   Chicken Rolls With Pesto

Preparation time: 20 minutes

Cooking time: 30 minutes

Servings: 1

Ingredients:

- Tablespoon pine nuts
- Yeast tablets
- Garlic cloves (chopped)
- Fresh basil
- Olive oil
- Chicken breast ready to slice:
- Preheat the oven to 175 ° C.
- Place the pine nuts in a dry pan and heat to a golden brown over medium heat for 3 minutes. Place on a plate and set aside.
- Place pine nuts, yeast flakes and garlic in a food processor and grind finely.
- Add basil and oil and mix briefly until you get pesto.

Direction:

1. Season with salt and pepper.
2. Place each piece of the chicken breast between 2 pieces of plastic wrap. 7 Roll in a frying pan or pasta until the chicken breasts grow out.
3. 0.6 cm thick.
4. Remove the plastic wrap, then apply pesto to the chicken.
5. Roll up the chicken breast and tie it with the cocktail skewers.
6. Season with salt and pepper.
7. Dissolve the coconut oil in the pan and use a high temperature to brown all sides of the chicken skin.
8. Place the chicken rolls on a baking sheet, place in the oven, and bake for 15 to 20 minutes, until cooked.
9. Slice it diagonally and serve it with other pesto sauce.

10. It was served with tomato salad.

Nutrition:

- Calories: 150
- Sodium: 33 mg
- Dietary Fiber: 1.6 g
- Total Fat: 4.3 g
- Total Carbs: 15.4 g
- Protein: 1.6 g

177.   Lemon Caper Pesto

Preparation time: 10 minutes

Servings: 1

Ingredients:

- 6 tablespoons fresh parsley leaves
- 3 cloves of garlic
- 2 tablespoons capers
- 2oz cashew nuts
- 2 tablespoons olive oil
- 1 tablespoon lemon juice
- Serves 8: 95 calories per serving

Directions:

1. Place all of the ingredients into a food processor and blitz until smooth.
2. Add a little extra oil if necessary.
3. Serve with pasta, vegetables or meat dishes.

Nutrition:

- Calories: 250
- Sodium: 32 mg
- Dietary Fiber: 1.6 g
- Total Fat: 4.1 g
- Total Carbs: 16.4 g
- Protein: 1.5 g

178.   Walnut & Mint Pesto

Preparation time: 10 minutes

Cooking time: 10 minutes

Servings: 1

Ingredients:

- 6 tablespoons fresh mint leaves
- 2oz walnuts
- 2 cloves of garlic
- 3½oz Parmesan cheese
- 1 tablespoon lemon juice

Direction:

1. Put all the ingredients into a food processor and;
2. Blend until it becomes a smooth paste.

Nutrition:

- Calories: 99
- Sodium: 33 mg
- Dietary Fiber: 1.6 g
- Total Fat: 4.4 g
- Total Carbs: 16.4 g
- Protein: 1.6 g

179.   Parsley Pesto

Preparation time: 10 minutes

Cooking time: 10 minutes

Servings: 1

Ingredients:

- 3oz Parmesan cheese, finely grated
- 2oz pine nuts
- 6 tablespoons fresh parsley leaves, chopped
- 2 cloves of garlic
- 2 tablespoons olive oil

Direction:

1. Put all of the ingredients into a food processor or blend until you have a smooth paste.

Nutrition:

- Calories: 104
- Sodium: 32 mg
- Dietary Fiber: 1.6 g
- Total Fat: 4.3 g
- Total Carbs: 16.2 g
- Protein: 1.3 g

Chapter 12:   Other Sirtfood Recipes

180.   Mustard

Preparation time: 20 minutes

Cooking time: 30 minutes

Servings: 1

Ingredients:

- Mustard seeds
- Water
- Apple cider vinegar
- 1 teaspoon lemon juice
- Honey
- 1/2 teaspoon dried turmeric

Directions:

1. Place mustard seeds, water and vinegar in a glass, cover and place in the refrigerator for 12 hours.
2. Put all the ingredients in a large measuring cup.
3. Use a hand blender to mix all the food.
4. Try mustard and add honey or salt.
5. Place mustard in a clean refrigerator for at least 3 weeks.

Nutrition:

- Calories: 360
- Sodium: 27 mg
- Dietary Fiber: 1.6 g
- Total Fat: 4.1 g
- Total Carbs: 12.3 g
- Protein: 1.3 g

181.   Bean Spread

Preparation time: 10 minutes

Cooking time: 7 hours

Servings: 4

Ingredients:

- 1 cup white beans, dried
- 1 teaspoon apple cider vinegar
- 1 cup veggie stock
- 1 tablespoon water

Directions:

1. In your slow cooker, mix beans with stock, stir, cover, cook on Low for 6 hours, drain, transfer to your food processor, add vinegar and water, pulse well, divide into bowls and serve.

Enjoy!

Nutrition:

- Calories: 181
- Sodium: 28 mg
- Dietary Fiber: 1.8 g
- Total Fat: 2.1 g
- Total Carbs: 1.3 g
- Protein: 4.1 g

182.   Carrots and Cauliflower Spread

Preparation time: 10 minutes

Cooking time: 40 minutes

Servings: 4

Ingredients:

- 1 cup carrots, sliced
- 2 cups cauliflower florets
- ½ cup cashews
- 2 and ½ cups water
- 1 cup almond milk
- 1 teaspoon garlic powder
- ¼ teaspoon smoked paprika

Directions:

1. In a small pot, mix the carrots with cauliflower, cashews and water, stir, cover, bring to a boil over medium heat, cook for 40 minutes, drain and transfer to a blender.
2. Add almond milk, garlic powder and paprika, pulse well, divide into small bowls and serve

Enjoy!

Nutrition:

- Calories 201
- Sodium: 38 mg
- Dietary Fiber: 1.3 g
- Total Fat: 2.1 g
- Total Carbs: 14.3 g
- Protein: 1.4 g

183.   Corn Spread

Preparation time: 10 minutes

Cooking time: 10 minutes

Servings: 6

Ingredients:

- 30 ounces canned corn, drained
- 2 green onions, chopped
- ½ cup coconut cream
- 1 jalapeno, chopped
- ½ teaspoon chili powder

Directions:

1. In a small pan, combine the corn with green onions, jalapeno and chili powder, stir, bring to a simmer, cook over medium heat for 10 minutes, leave aside to cool down, add coconut cream, stir well, divide into small bowls and serve as a spread.

Enjoy!

Nutrition:

- Calories: 192
- Sodium: 33 mg
- Dietary Fiber: 1.4 g
- Total Fat: 4.1 g
- Total Carbs: 14.3 g
- Protein: 1.2 g

184.   Mussels in Red Wine Sauce

Preparation time: 5 minutes

Cooking time: 5 minutes

Servings: 2

Ingredients:

- 800g mussels
- 2 x 400g tins of chopped tomatoes
- 25g butter
- 1 fresh chives, chopped
- 1 fresh parsley, chopped
- 1 bird's-eye chili, finely chopped
- 4 cloves of garlic, crushed
- 400mls red wine
- Juice of 1 lemon

Directions:

1. Wash the mussels, remove their beards and set them aside.
2. Heat the butter in a large saucepan and add in the red wine.
3. Reduce the heat and add the parsley, chives, chili and garlic whilst stirring.
4. Add in the tomatoes, lemon juice and mussels.
5. Cover the saucepan and cook for 2-3.
6. Remove the saucepan from the heat and take out any mussels which haven't opened and discard them.
7. Serve and eat immediately.

Nutrition:

- Calories: 364
- Net carbs: 3.3g
- Fat: 4.9g
- Fiber: 0.7g

- Protein: 8.2g

185.   Roast Balsamic Vegetables

Preparation time: 10 minutes

Cooking time: 45 minutes

Servings: 4

Ingredients:

- 4 tomatoes, chopped
- 2 red onions, chopped
- 3 sweet potatoes, peeled and chopped
- 100g red chicory (or if unavailable, use yellow)
- 100g kale, finely chopped
- 300g potatoes, peeled and chopped
- 5 stalks of celery, chopped
- 1 bird's-eye chili, de-seeded and finely chopped
- 2g fresh parsley, chopped
- 2gs fresh coriander (cilantro) chopped
- 3 teaspoons olive oil
- 2 teaspoons balsamic vinegar
- 1 teaspoon mustard
- Sea salt
- Freshly ground black pepper

Directions:

1. Place the olive oil, balsamic, mustard, parsley and coriander (cilantro) into a bowl and mix well.
2. Toss all the remaining ingredients into the dressing and season with salt and pepper.
3. Transfer the vegetables to an ovenproof dish and cook in the oven at 200C/400F for 45 minutes.

Nutrition:

- Calories: 310
- Net carbs: 1.1g
- Fiber: 0.2g
- Protein: 0.2g

186.   Tomato and Goat's Pizza

Preparation time: 15 minutes

Cooking time: 20 minutes

Servings: 2

Ingredients:

- 225g buckwheat flour
- 2 teaspoons dried yeast
- Pinch of salt
- 150mls slightly water
- 1 teaspoon olive oil
- For the Topping:
- 75g feta cheese, crumbled
- 75g peseta (or tomato paste)
- 1 tomato, sliced
- 1 red onion, finely chopped
- 25g rocket (arugula) leaves, chopped

Directions:

1. In a bowl, combine all the ingredients for the pizza dough then allow it to stand for at least an hour until it has doubled in size.
2. Roll the dough out to a size to suit you.
3. Spoon the passata onto the base and add the rest of the toppings.
4. Bake in the oven at 200C/400F for 15-20 minutes or until browned at the edges and crispy and serve.

Nutrition:

- Calories: 585
- Net carbs: 77g
- Fat: 8.1g
- Fiber: 7.6g
- Protein: 22.9g

187.   Tender Spiced Lamb

Preparation time: 20 minutes

Cooking time: 4 hours 20 minutes

Servings: 8

Ingredients:

- 1.35kg lamb shoulder
- 3 red onions, sliced
- 3 cloves of garlic, crushed
- 1 bird's eye chili, finely chopped
- 1 teaspoon turmeric
- 1 teaspoon ground cumin
- ½ teaspoon ground coriander (cilantro)
- ¼ teaspoon ground cinnamon
- 2 tablespoons olive oil

Directions:

1. In a bowl, combine the chili, garlic and spices with olive oil.
2. Coat the lamb with the spice mixture and marinate it for an hour, or overnight if you can.
3. Heat the remaining oil in a pan, add the lamb and brown it for 3-4 minutes on all sides to seal it.
4. Place the lamb in an ovenproof dish.
5. Add in the red onions and cover the dish with foil.
6. Transfer to the oven and roast at 170C/325F for 4 hours. The lamb should be extremely tender and falling off the bone.
7. Serve with rice or couscous, salad or vegetables.

Nutrition:

- Calories: 455
- Net carbs: 28g

- Fat: 9.8g
- Fiber: 11g
- Protein: 20g

188. Chili Cod Fillets

Preparation time: 10 minutes

Cooking time: 10 minutes

Servings: 4

Ingredients:

- 4 cod fillets each)
- 2 teaspoons fresh parsley, chopped
- 2 bird's-eye chilies (or more if you like it hot)
- 2 cloves of garlic, chopped
- 4 teaspoons olive oil

Directions:

1. Heat a of olive oil in a frying pan, add the fish and cook for 7-8 minutes or until thoroughly cooked, turning once halfway through.
2. Remove and keep warm.
3. Pour the remaining olive oil into the pan and add the chili, chopped garlic and parsley.
4. Warm it thoroughly.
5. Serve the fish onto plates and pour the warm chili oil over it.

Nutrition:

- Calories: 246
- Net carbs: 5.5g
- Fat: 0.5g
- Fiber: 0.7g
- Protein: 18.5g

189.   Steak and Mushroom Noodles

Preparation time: 10 minutes

Cooking time: 20 minutes

Servings: 4

Ingredients:

- 100g shitake mushrooms, halved, if large
- 100g chestnut mushrooms, sliced
- 150g udon noodles
- 75g kale, finely chopped
- 75g baby leaf spinach, chopped
- 2 sirloin steaks
- 2 teaspoons miso paste
- 2.5cm piece fresh ginger, finely chopped
- 2 teaspoons olive oil
- 1 star anise
- 1 red chili, finely sliced
- 1 red onion, finely chopped
- 1 fresh coriander (cilantro) chopped
- 1 liter (1½ pints) warm water

Directions:

1. Pour the water into a saucepan and add in the miso, star anise and ginger.
2. Bring it to the boil, reduce the heat and simmer gently.
3. In the meantime, cook the noodles according to their instructions then drain them.
4. Heat the oil in a saucepan, add the steak and cook for around 2-3 minutes on each side (or 1-2 minutes, for rare meat).
5. Remove the meat and set aside.
6. Place the mushrooms, spinach, coriander (cilantro) and kale into the miso broth and cook for 5 minutes.

7. In the meantime, heat the remaining oil in a separate pan and fry the chili and onion for 4 minutes, until softened.
8. Serve the noodles into bowls and pour the soup on top.
9. Thinly slice the steaks and add them to the top.
10. Serve immediately.

Nutrition:

- Calories: 296
- Net carbs: 24.6g
- Fat: 13.7g
- Fiber: 0.7g
- Protein: 32.9g

190.   Masala Scallops

Preparation time: 10 minutes

Cooking time: 20 minutes

Servings: 4

Ingredients:

- 2 tablespoons olive oil
- 2 jalapenos, chopped
- 1 pound sea scallops
- A pinch of salt and black pepper
- ¼ teaspoon cinnamon powder
- 1 teaspoon garam masala
- 1 teaspoon coriander, ground
- 1 teaspoon cumin, ground
- 2 tablespoons cilantro, chopped

Directions:

1. Heat up a pan with the oil over medium heat, add the jalapenos, cinnamon and the other ingredients except the scallops and cook for 10 minutes.
2. Add the rest of the ingredients, toss, cook for 10 minutes more, divide into bowls and serve.

Nutrition:

- Calories: 251
- Fat: 4g
- Fiber: 4g
- Carbs: 11g
- Protein: 17g

191.   Sirtfood Breakfast Scramble

So delicious! A great way to start your morning!

Preparation time: 5 minutes

Cooking time: 0 minutes

Servings: 1

Ingredients:

- 1 teaspoon ground turmeric
- 2 eggs
- 1/3 oz. parsley, finely chopped
- 1 teaspoon mild curry powder
- ¼ cup kale, roughly chopped
- 1 handful of button mushrooms, thinly sliced
- 1 teaspoon extra virgin olive oil
- ½ bird's eye chili, thinly sliced

Directions:

1. Mix the turmeric and curry powder and add a little water until you have reached a light paste.
2. Steam the kale for 2-3 minutes.
3. Heat the oil in a frying pan over a medium heat and fry the chili and mushrooms for 2-3 minutes until they have started to brown and soften.
4. Add the eggs and spice paste and cook over a medium heat, then add the kale and continue to cook for a further minute.
5. Finally, add the parsley, mix well and enjoy!

Nutrition:

- Calories 268,
- Fat 21g,
- Carbohydrates 13g,
- Protein 10g

192. Tuna and Tomatoes

Preparation time: 5 minutes

Cooking time: 20 minutes

Servings: 4

Ingredients:

- 1 yellow onion, chopped
- 1 tablespoon olive oil
- 1 pound tuna fillets, boneless, skinless and cubed
- 1 cup tomatoes, chopped
- 1 red pepper, chopped
- 1 teaspoon sweet paprika
- 1 tablespoon coriander, chopped

Directions:

1. Heat up a pan with the oil over medium heat, add the onions and the pepper and cook for 5 minutes.
2. Add the fish and the other ingredients, cook everything for 15 minutes, divide between plates and serve.

Nutrition:

- Calories: 215
- Fat: 4g
- Fiber: 7g
- Carbs: 14g
- Protein: 7g

193. Lemongrass and Ginger Mackerel

Preparation time: 10 minutes

Cooking time: 25 minutes

Servings: 4

Ingredients:

- 4 mackerel fillets, skinless and boneless
- 2 tablespoons olive oil
- 1 tablespoon ginger, grated
- 2 lemongrass sticks, chopped
- 2 red chilies, chopped
- Juice of 1 lime
- A handful parsley, chopped

Directions:

1. In a roasting pan, combine the mackerel with the oil, ginger and the other ingredients, toss and bake at 390 degrees F for 25 minutes.
2. Divide everything between plates and serve.

Nutrition:

- Calories: 251
- Fat: 3g
- Fiber: 4g
- Carbs: 14g
- Protein: 8g

194.   Scallops with Almonds and Mushrooms

Preparation time: 5 minutes

Cooking time: 10 minutes

Servings: 4

Ingredients:

- 1 pound scallops
- 2 tablespoons olive oil
- 4 scallions, chopped
- A pinch of salt and black pepper
- ½ cup mushrooms, sliced
- 2 tablespoon almonds, chopped
- 1 cup coconut cream

Directions:

1. Heat up a pan with the oil over medium heat; add the scallions and the mushrooms and sauté for 2 minutes.
2. Add the scallops and the other ingredients, toss, cook over medium heat for 8 minutes more, divide into bowls and serve.

Nutrition:

- Calories: 322
- Fat: 23.7g
- Fiber: 2.2g
- Carbs: 8.1g
- Protein: 21.6g

195.   Scallops and Sweet Potatoes

Preparation time: 5 minutes

Cooking time: 22 minutes

Servings: 4

Ingredients:

- 1 pound scallops
- ½ teaspoon rosemary, dried
- ½ teaspoon oregano, dried
- 2 tablespoons avocado oil
- 1 yellow onion, chopped
- 2 sweet potatoes, peeled and cubed
- ½ cup chicken stock
- 1 tablespoon cilantro, chopped
- A pinch of salt and black pepper

Directions:

1. Heat up a pan with the oil over medium heat; add the onion and sauté for 2 minutes.
2. Add the sweet potatoes and the stock, toss and cook for 10 minutes more.
3. Add the scallops and the remaining ingredients, toss, cook for another 10 minutes, divide everything into bowls and serve.

Nutrition:

- Calories: 211
- Fat: 2g
- Fiber: 4.1g
- Carbs: 26.9g
- Protein: 20.7g

196.   Rosemary Endives

Preparation time: 10 minutes

Cooking time: 0 minutes

Servings: 4

Ingredients:

- 2 tablespoons olive oil
- 1tablespoon dried rosemary
- 2 halved endives
- ¼ tablespoon black pepper
- ½ tablespoon turmeric powder

Directions:

1. In a baking pan, combine the endives with the oil and the other ingredients, toss gently, introduce in the oven and bake at 400F for 20 minutes.
2. Divide between plates and serve.

Nutrition:

- Calories: 66
- Fat: 7.1g
- Carbs: 1.2 g
- Protein: 0.3g
- Sugars: 1.3g
- Sodium: 113mg

197.   Flax Waffles

Preparation Time: 5 minutes

Cooking Time: 5 minutes

Servings: 2

Ingredients:

- ½ cup whole-wheat flour
- 1/3 tablespoon flaxseed meal
- ½ teaspoon baking powder
- 1 tablespoon olive oil
- ½ cup almond milk, unsweetened
- Extra:
- ¼ teaspoon vanilla extract, unsweetened
- 2 tablespoons coconut sugar

Directions

1. Switch on a minute's waffle maker and let it preheat for 5 minutes.
2. Meanwhile, take a medium bowl, place all the ingredients in it, and then mix by using an immersion blender until smooth.
3. Ladle the batter evenly into the waffle maker, shut with lid, and let it cook for 3 to 4 minutes until firm and golden brown.
4. Serve straight away.

Nutrition:

- Calories 180
- Fats 8.6 g
- Protein 4.1 g
- Carbs 21.7 g
- Fiber 3.7 g

198.   Prawn Arrabbiata

Preparation Time: 10 minutes

Cooking Time: 25 minutes

Servings: 2

Ingredients:

- 125-150 g Raw or cooked prawns (Ideally ruler prawns)
- 65 g Buckwheat pasta
- 1 tbsp. extra virgin olive oil
- For Arrabbiata sauce
- 40 g Red onion, finely slashed
- 1 Garlic clove, finely slashed
- 30 g Celery, finely slashed
- 1 Bird's eye bean stew, finely hacked
- 1 tsp. Dried blended herbs
- 1 tsp. extra virgin olive oil
- 2tbsps. White wine (discretionary)
- 400 g Tinned slashed tomatoes
- 1 tbsp. Chopped parsley

Directions:

1. Fry the onion, garlic, celery and bean stew and dried herbs in the oil over a medium-low warmth for 1–2 minutes.
2. Turn the heat up to medium, include the wine and cook for one moment.
3. Include the tomatoes and leave the sauce to stew over a medium-low warmth for 20–30 minutes, until it has a pleasant creamy consistency.
4. On the off chance that you feel the sauce is getting too thick just include a little water.
5. While the sauce is cooking, carry a container of water to the bubble and cook the pasta as per the bundle guidelines.
6. At the point when prepared just as you would prefer, channel, hurl with the olive oil and keep in the container until required.

7. On the off that you are utilizing crude prawns mix them to the sauce and bake for a further 3–4 minutes until it has turned pink and dark, including the parsley and serve.
8. If you are utilizing cooked prawns, include them with the parsley, carry the sauce to the bubble and help.
9. Add pasta to the sauce, blend altogether yet tenderly and serve.

Nutrition:

- 15 calories
- 30 g complete fat
- 1.2 g immersed fat
- 25 mg cholesterol
- 20 mg sodium
- 93 mg potassium
- 2g starches
- 70 mcg folate
- 15 mg calcium
- 57 mg magnesium

199.   Cabbage with Coconut & Turnip

Preparation Time: 10 minutes

Cooking Time: 10 minutes

Servings: 2

Ingredients:

- 1 lb. unpeeled and halved turnips
- 2tbsps. coconut oil
- 1 pinch Asafetida
- 1 tsp. black mustard seeds
- 1 tsp. cumin seeds
- 2 dried red chilies
- 1 fresh seedless and thinly sliced red or green chili
- 1 finely shredded cabbage head
- 1/2 Seville orange juice
- 2tbsps. desiccated or shaved fresh coconut

Directions:

1. In a large pot, pour in water with salt then boil it.
2. Add the potatoes then stir.
3. Cook for about 10 minutes.
4. Drain the water then them to a bowl.
5. Crush the potatoes with a fork gently.
6. In a skillet, heat the oil then add spices, the chilies, and Asafetida.
7. Sauté for about 2 minutes then toss in salt, fresh chili, and the cabbage.
8. Stir as you cook it for about 4 minutes.
9. Stir in the drained potatoes then cook for 3 minutes.
10. Add in the Seville orange juice, coriander, and coconut.
11. Properly mix them.
12. Serve warm with coconut yogurt.

Nutrition:

- Calories: 604 kcal
- Fat: 30.6g
- Carbs: 21.4g
- Protein: 54.6g

200.   Turmeric & Lemon Dressing

Preparation time: 10 minutes

Cooking time: 30 minutes

Servings: 1

Ingredients

- 1 teaspoon turmeric
- 4 tablespoons olive oil
- Juice of 1 lemon

Directions

1. Combine all the ingredients in bowl and serve with salads.
2. Eat straight away.

Nutrition:

- Calories: 125,
- Sodium: 32 mg,
- Dietary Fibre: 1.6 g,
- Total Fat: 3.3 g,
- Total Carbs: 16.3 g,
- Protein: 1.5 g.

201. Vinaigrette

Preparation time: 10 minutes

Cooking time: 10 minutes

Servings: 2

Ingredients:

- A teaspoon of yellow mustard
- A spoon of white wine vinegar
- 1 Teaspoon of honey
- 165 ml of prepared olive oil:

Directions

1. Mix mustard, vinegar and honey in a bowl.
2. Add a small amount of olive oil and stir until the vinegar thickens.
3. Season with salt and pepper.

Nutrition:

- Calories: 1495
- Sodium: 33 mg
- Dietary Fibre: 1.4 g
- Total Fat: 4.3 g
- Total Carbs: 16.2 g
- Protein: 1.5 g

202.   Walnut Vinaigrette

Preparation time: 10 minutes

Cooking time: 10 minutes

Servings: 1

Ingredients:

- 1 clove garlic, finely chopped
- 6 tablespoons olive oil
- 3 tablespoons red wine vinegar
- 1 tablespoon walnut oil
- Sea salt
- Freshly ground black pepper

Directions:

1. Combine all of the ingredients in a bowl or container and season with salt and pepper.
2. Use immediately or store in the fridge.

Nutrition:

- Calories: 109
- Sodium: 33 mg
- Dietary Fibre: 1.6 g
- Total Fat: 4.3 g
- Total Carbs: 16.4 g
- Protein: 1.6 g

203.   Garlic Vinaigrette

Preparation time: 10 minutes

Cooking time: 30 minutes

Servings: 1

Ingredients

- 1 clove garlic, crushed
- 4 tablespoons olive oil
- 1 tablespoon lemon juice
- Freshly ground black pepper

Directions

1. Simply mix all of the ingredients together.
2. It can either be stored or used straight away.

Nutrition:

- Calories: 104
- Sodium: 35 mg
- Dietary Fibre: 1.3 g
- Total Fat: 3.1 g
- Total Carbs: 16.2 g
- Protein: 1.3 g

204.   Teriyaki Sauce

Preparation time: 10 minutes

Cooking time: 30 minutes

Servings: 1

Ingredients

- 7fl oz soy sauce
- 7fl oz pineapple juice
- 1 teaspoon red wine vinegar
- 1-inch chunk of fresh ginger root, peeled and chopped
- 2 cloves of garlic

Directions

1. Place the ingredients into a saucepan, bring them to the boil, reduce the heat and simmer for 10 minutes.
2. Let it cool then remove the garlic and ginger.
3. Store it in a container in the fridge until ready to use.
4. Use as a marinade for meat, fish and tofu dishes.

Nutrition:

- Calories: 267
- Sodium: 33 mg
- Dietary Fibre: 1.2g
- Total Fat: 4.3 g
- Total Carbs: 16.2 g
- Protein: 1.3 g

205. Sweet And Sour Sauce

Preparation time: 10 minutes

Cooking time: 10 minutes

Servings: 1

Ingredients:

- Apple cider vinegar
- 1/2 tablespoon tomato paste
- A teaspoon of coconut amino acid
- Bamboo spoon
- Water treatment
- Chopped vegetables.

Directions:

1. Mix kudzu powder with five tablespoons of cold water to make a paste.
2. Then put all the other spices in the pot, then add the kudzu paste.
3. Melt coconut oil in a pan and fry onions.
4. Add green pepper, cabbage, cabbage and bean sprouts, then cook until the vegetables are tender.
5. Add pineapple and cashew nuts and mix a few times.
6. Just pour a little spice into the pot.

Nutrition:

- Calories: 495
- Sodium: 33 mg
- Dietary Fibre: 1.4 g
- Total Fat: 4.5 g
- Total Carbs: 16.5 g
- Protein: 1.7 g

206.   Italian Veggie Salsa

Preparation time: 10 minutes

Cooking time: 10 minutes

Servings: 4

Ingredients:

- 2 red bell peppers, cut into medium wedges
- 3 zucchinis, sliced
- ½ cup garlic, minced
- 2 tablespoons olive oil
- A pinch of black pepper
- 1 teaspoon Italian seasoning

Directions:

1. Heat up a pan with the oil over medium-high heat, add bell peppers and zucchini, toss and cook for 5 minutes.
2. Add garlic, black pepper and Italian seasoning, toss, cook for 5 minutes more, divide into small cups and serve as a snack.

Enjoy!

Nutrition:

- Calories 132
- Sodium: 33 mg
- Dietary Fibre: 2.4 g
- Total Fat: 4.2 g
- Total Carbs: 14.3 g
- Protein: 1.5 g

207.   The Salsa

Preparation time: 20 minutes

Cooking time: 40 minutes

Servings: 1

Ingredients

- One small tomato
- One Thai chili, thinly sliced.
- One teaspoon of caper, fine cut
- Parsley - 2 teaspoons fine cut
- 1/4 of a lemon's juice

Directions

1. Remove the eye from the tomato to make the salsa and slice it finely, ensuring that the fluid remains in as much as possible.
2. Combine Chile, capers, lemon juice and parsley. You might mix it all in, but the end product is a little different.
3. Oven to 220 degrees Celsius (425 ° F), in one teaspoon, marinate the chicken breast with a little oil and lemon juice.
4. Leave for five to ten minutes.
5. Then add the marinated chicken and cook on either side for about a minute, until pale golden, transfer to the oven (on a baking tray, if your pan is not ovenproof), 8 to 10 minutes or until cooked.
6. Remove from the oven, cover with tape, and wait until eaten for five minutes.
7. Cook the kale for 5 minutes in a steamer in the meantime, add a little butter, fry the red onions and the ginger and then mix in the fluffy but not browned mix.
8. Cook the buckwheat with the remaining teaspoon of turmeric according to the package instructions.
9. Eat rice, tomatoes and salsa. Eat together.

Nutrition:

- Calories: 104
- Sodium: 33 mg
- Dietary Fibre: 1.6 g
- Total Fat: 4.3 g
- Total Carbs: 15.3 g
- Protein: 1.3 g

208.   Eggplant Salsa

Preparation time: 10 minutes

Cooking time: 10 minutes

Servings: 4

Ingredients:

- 1 and ½ cups tomatoes, chopped
- 3 cups eggplant, cubed
- A drizzle of olive oil
- 2 teaspoons capers
- 6 ounces of green olives, pitted and sliced
- 4 garlic cloves, minced
- 2 teaspoons balsamic vinegar
- 1 tablespoon basil, chopped
- Black pepper to the taste

Directions:

1. Heat up a pan with the oil over medium-high heat, add eggplant, stir and cook for 5 minutes.
2. Add tomatoes, capers, olives, garlic, vinegar, basil and black pepper, toss, cook for 5 minutes more, divide into small cups and serve cold.

Enjoy!

Nutrition:

- Calories: 120
- Sodium: 24 mg
- Dietary Fibre: 1.8 g
- Total Fat: 2.1 g
- Total Carbs: 1.8 g
- Protein: 1.8 g

209.   Mung Sprouts Salsa

Preparation time: 10 minutes

Cooking time: 0 minutes

Servings: 2

Ingredients:

- 1 red onion, chopped
- 2 cups mung beans, sprouted
- A pinch of red chili powder
- 1 green chili pepper, chopped
- 1 tomato, chopped
- 1 teaspoon chaat masala
- 1 teaspoon lemon juice
- 1 tablespoon coriander, chopped
- Black pepper to the taste

Directions:

1. In a salad bowl, mix onion with mung sprouts, chili pepper, tomato, chili powder, chaat masala, lemon juice, coriander and pepper, toss well, divide into small cups and serve.

Enjoy!

Nutrition:

- Calories: 100
- Sodium: 23 mg
- Dietary Fibre: 1.4 g
- Total Fat: 2.1 g
- Total Carbs: 10.3 g
- Protein: 1.2 g

210.   Black Bean Salsa

Preparation time: 10 minutes

Cooking time: 0 minutes

Servings: 6

Ingredients:

- 1 tablespoon coconut aminos
- ½ teaspoon cumin, ground
- 1 cup canned black beans, no-salt-added, drained and rinsed
- 1 cup salsa
- 6 cups romaine lettuce leaves, torn
- ½ cup avocado, peeled, pitted and cubed

Directions:

1. In a bowl, combine the beans with the aminos, cumin, salsa, lettuce and avocado, toss, divide into small bowls and serve as a snack.

Enjoy!

Nutrition:

- Calories: 181
- Sodium: 33 mg
- Dietary Fibre: 1.4 g
- Total Fat: 3.1 g
- Total Carbs: 14.3 g
- Protein: 1.2 g

211. Salsa Bean Dip

Preparation time: 10 minutes

Cooking time: 20 minutes

Servings: 6

Ingredients:

- ½ cup salsa
- 2 cups canned white beans, no-salt-added, drained and rinsed
- 1 cup low-fat cheddar, shredded
- 2 tablespoons green onions, chopped

Directions:

1. In a small pot, combine the beans with the green onions and salsa, stir, bring to a simmer over medium heat, cook for 20 minutes, add cheese, stir until it melts, take off heat, leave aside to cool down, divide into bowls and serve.

Enjoy!

Nutrition:

- Calories: 212
- Sodium: 32 mg
- Dietary Fibre: 1.4 g
- Total Fat: 2.1 g
- Total Carbs: 12.3 g
- Protein: 1.5 g

212. Rosemary Squash Dip

Preparation time: 10 minutes

Cooking time: 40 minutes

Servings: 4

Ingredients:

- 1 cup butternut squash, peeled and cubed
- 1 tablespoon water
- Cooking spray
- 2 tablespoons coconut milk
- 2 teaspoons rosemary, dried
- Black pepper to the taste

Directions:

1. Spread squash cubes on a lined baking sheet, spray some cooking oil, introduce in the oven, bake at 365 degrees F for 40 minutes, transfer to your blender, add water, milk, rosemary and black pepper, pulse well, divide into small bowls and serve.

Enjoy!

Nutrition:

- Calories: 182
- Sodium: 27 mg
- Dietary Fibre: 1.4 g
- Total Fat: 2.1 g
- Total Carbs: 7.3 g
- Protein: 1.6 g

213.   Sesame Dip

Preparation time: 10 minutes

Cooking time: 0 minutes

Servings: 6

Ingredients:

- 1 cup sesame seed paste, pure
- Black pepper to the taste
- 1 cup veggie stock
- ½ cup lemon juice
- ½ teaspoon cumin, ground
- 3 garlic cloves, chopped

Directions:

1. In your food processor, mix the sesame paste with black pepper, stock, lemon juice, cumin and garlic, pulse very well, divide into bowls and serve as a party dip.

Enjoy!

Nutrition:

- Calories: 120
- Sodium: 26 mg
- Dietary Fibre: 1.8 g
- Total Fat: 2.1 g
- Total Carbs: 11.4 g
- Protein: 1.9 g

214.   Mushroom Dip

Preparation time: 10 minutes

Cooking time: 20 minutes

Servings: 6

Ingredients:

- 1 cup yellow onion, chopped
- 3 garlic cloves, minced
- 1-pound mushrooms, chopped
- 28 ounces tomato sauce, no-salt-added
- Black pepper to the taste

Directions:

1. Put the onion in a pot, add garlic, mushrooms, black pepper and tomato sauce, stir, cook over medium heat for 20 minutes, leave aside to cool down, divide into small bowls and serve.

   Enjoy!

Nutrition:

- Calories 215
- Sodium: 34 mg
- Dietary Fibre: 1.3 g
- Total Fat: 4.3 g
- Total Carbs: 16.6
- Protein: 1.4 g

Conclusion

Thank you for making it to the end. Despite the early stage of the Sirtfood juicing and fasting diet seems just ideal for those who may want to quickly lose some weight, the Sirtfood diet's over-riding goal is to include healthy food in your diet to improve your well-being and immune system. There is, however, a more important target. While the first seven days can seem very challenging, the longer-term approach will work for anyone.

You can continue the fat burning while enjoying your regular favorites by focusing on introducing Sirtfood rich ingredients into your daily meals. This is an eating program that will continue to provide benefits for a long period of time.

A heavy emphasis on sirtfoods, supplemented by protein-rich animal products and omega-3 fish sources, offers the benefits of sirtuin activation and the full range of vital nutrients. Like any diet, however, the Sirtfood Diet will not be able to meet the requirements of selenium and vitamin D, and it is suggested that it be supplemented. For those who are after a vegan or vegetarian regime, certain nutrients should be considered too. Periodic exercise also induces full activation of the sirtuin.

At the end of this book, if you want to reap Sirtfoods' stunning results, here are some suggested ways to start your diet:

Security first-Contact your healthcare professional, particularly if you have a current illness before beginning some new diet or routine. This should guarantee that the plan will not harm any medication you might be taking or negatively impact your safety. Do not worry; the diet on Sirtfood is pretty healthy.

Knowledge is power-This diet is still brand new, but there is still plenty of information available, and much more upcoming as this diet is gaining popularity quickly. You can also search the web for recipes, food alternatives, nutritional value, and much more.

Follow the guidelines-Sirtfood is guaranteed to deliver results, if and only if you follow the diet guide carefully and the food suggested.

Start a physical exercise-Sirtfood diet that can actually burn those fats and gain strength, but I suggest you start trying to add physical activity to your regular activities. A 30-minute stroll a day will do your body good and would also monitor the effects easily. Additionally, by exercise like avoiding and fighting health problems, helping change your mindset, encouraging healthier sleep, losing calories, offering you an extra boost, and more, there are other wonderful results.

Help yourself-You can start by removing processed as well as starchy food from your regular diet aside from obeying what is permitted in the food program. Stop junk eating! It can monitor Sirtfood Diet performance easily.

Be comfortable for the initial "restrictions" - Obviously, if you want to achieve better outcomes, you need to "sacrifice" a little to get the maximum advantages of a Sirtfood diet. But don't worry, the first 3 days are only the toughest for this diet as it will involve calorie restrictions, but be assured it'll become easier every day. Despite the constraints imposed for those who attempted the diet wasn't that tough for them, the explanation is meal preparation carefully. When you chose carefully, you won't go hungry on this plan.

Hit the grocery store-Sirtfood diet based on certain foods. Those foods were selected because of their ability to sirtuin trigger. And if you don't obey the chart, then you're not going to get results. Do not panic, because I will provide a list of suggested food items; Plus, there is no excessively expensive type of food, and you can discover it readily available just about anywhere (you might just have some hidden in your refrigerator already).

Incorporate a diet partner-This diet could also benefit greatly your partner, family, or friends (not just overweight persons), plus it's easier to remember, share recipes with, or even prepare meals dishes when you have an organized approach.

Plan your meals accordingly-Preparing your meals are a huge aid whatever plan you might be on. You will still take the opportunity to assess the options and fill up the cupboard, not only does that will the burden from dieting. You have to adopt a calorie count for the first half of this plan. You'll be amazed that many loading dishes are permitted with fewer calories and filled with sirtuins.

Be good to yourself - Don't raise goals too high. Yes, some can quickly lose 7 pounds a week, but understand that not all of our bodies are the same; and your strong commitment would also count, of course. Other factors may be the inclusion in the diet schedule of an activity routine and might allow the cycle of losing weight quickly.

Document your improvement-You can begin by taking the pictures "before" and taking the appropriate body composition. You should even maintain a diet log and monitor your meal intake. Every week or process notes improvements in the body. You should also provide several targets to drive you on more with the diet.

I hope you have learned something and good luck on your sirtfood journey!

Did you enjoy this cookbook?

If you enjoyed this book, it would be awesome if you could leave a quick review on Amazon. Your feedback is much appreciated and I would love to hear from you.

<u>Leave a Review on Amazon</u>

Thanks so much!!